Skills Training Manual for
Treating Borderline Personality Disorder

DIAGNOSIS AND TREATMENT OF MENTAL DISORDERS
Allen Frances, MD, *Series Editor*

Skills Training Manual for Treating Borderline Personality Disorder

Marsha M. Linehan, Ph.D.
University of Washington

THE GUILFORD PRESS
New York   London

©1993 The Guilford Press
A Division of Guilford Publications, Inc.
72 Spring Street, New York, NY 10012

Printed in the United States of America

This book is printed on acid-free paper.

Last digit is print number: 9   8   7   6   5   4

Library of Congress Cataloging-in-Publication Data

Linehan, Marsha.
    Skills training manual for treating borderline personality
disorder / Marsha M. Linehan.
       p.   cm.—(Diagnosis and treatment of mental disorders)
    Includes bibliographical references and index.
    ISBN 0-89862-034-1
    1. Borderline personality disorder—Treatment.   2. Social skills-
-Study and teaching.   3. Group psychotherapy.   I. Title.
II. Series.
    [DNLM: 1. Borderline Personality Disorder—therapy—handbooks.
WM 39 L754s 1993]
RC569.5.B67L563   1993
616.85'85206—dc20
DNLM/DLC
for Library of Congress   93-20483
                                                       CIP

To my teachers,
Gerald C. Davison, Ph.D.,
and
Willigis Jäger, O.S.B. (Ko-un Roshi).
Each taught me "skillful means."

Preface

This manual has been evolving for the past 20 or so years. The version presented here is the latest of dozens of versions prepared over the years (and the first of many more versions likely to result from further experience). The specific skills and client handouts have been "road-tested" with over 100 clients in several settings. However, each new group of clients seems to find at least one area of the skills training program to criticize and improve. Thus, revisions have been made almost continually. In a similar fashion, the user of this manual should feel free to modify, shorten, lengthen, and/or reorganize the modules described here.

I considered developing a shortened version of these skills (e.g., 10 lessons) for use in acute care settings. Each lesson would revolve around one or more of the client handouts and associated homework sheets. A number of acute care psychiatric inpatient units have already done this to meet their own needs. Looking at the various shortened versions, I have been struck by the diversity of how different units have accomplished this. Some units offer only the distress tolerance and core mindfulness skills modules, covering these in 8 or 10 daily sessions. Others have selected two or three handouts from each skills module. Still others have selected a few from the emotion regulation and distress tolerance modules and then added a few skills handouts from other treatment packages. I believe that there is probably no one best set of only 10 lessons. Instead, I encourage the interested user of this manual to experiment with various sets of shortened versions.

Acknowledgments

Much of what is in this manual I learned from the many clients who participated in skills training groups that I have conducted over the years. I am grateful to all those who put up with the many versions that did not work or were not useful, and to those among them who gave enough feedback for me to make needed revisions in the skills being taught.

Much of the improvement and fine-tuning of the therapist strategies used to teach skills, especially in a group setting, came from the clinical wisdom of my cotherapists over the years: Douglas Allmon, Ph.D., Beatriz Aramburu, Ph.D., Hugh Armstrong, Ph.D., Katherine Draper, Alan Fruzzetti, Ph.D., Mary Ann Goodwyn, Ph.D., Heidi Heard, Gerald Hover, Ph.D., Connie Kehrer, Walter Kuciej, Maxine Lillie, Kay Olheiser, Wendy Pava, Edward Shearin, Ph.D., Darren Tutek, Amy Wagner, Jennifer Waltz, and Elizabeth Wasson. When I first started teaching therapists how to conduct skills training with borderline patients, I had little idea of the actual strategies needed to accomplish this task. My cotherapists were models of patience and perseverance through many attempts on my part to organize the strategies, taken from the companion text to this manual, in a coherent and useful fashion.

My research team and colleagues over the years—John Chiles, M.D., Kelly Egan, Ph.D., Heidi Heard, Andre Ivanoff, Ph.D., Connie Kehrer, Joan Lockard, Ph.D., Steve McCutcheon, Ph.D., Evelyn Mercier, Steve Nelson, Ph.D., Kirk Strosahl, Ph.D., and Darren Tutek—have been invaluable in providing the support and many of the ideas that have nourished the development of an empirically grounded treatment for borderline personality disorder. It was the empirical data showing the effectiveness as a whole of dialectical behavior therapy that prompted me to write this manual. The research team produced those data.

The final draft of the manual was written while I was on sabbatical at Cornell Medical Center/New York Hospital in White Plains, New York. While I was there, Charles Swensen, M.D., and his staff were implementing these skills training modules on the inpatient unit for borderline patients. I revised my modules yet again, learning from them better ways to organize the materials and teach them to the borderline population. Leslie Horton, my secretary on the treatment research project, and Chihae Yun also deserve much of the credit for organizing me and the materials that later constituted this book.

Development and writing of this treatment manual were partially supported by Grant

No. MH34486 from the National Institute of Mental Health. Morris Parloff, Ph.D., Irene Elkin, Ph.D., Barry Wolfe, Ph.D., and Tracie Shea, Ph.D., nurtured and fought for this work from the beginning, and deserve much of the credit for the success of the research on which this treatment approach is based.

Last, but certainly not least, I want to thank my copy editor, Marie Sprayberry, the Managing Editor, Rowena Howells, and the staff at The Guilford Press. In getting this manual out in a timely fashion they each had occasion to practice all the distress tolerence skills in this book. Their concern for this manuscript and this form of treatment was evident at every step.

Contents

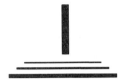

Rationale for Psychosocial Skills Training with Borderline Clients[1]

Individuals meeting criteria for borderline personality disorder (BPD) are flooding mental health and clinical practitioners' offices. Even when potentially effective pharmacotherapy is instituted, it is commonly assumed that psychosocial treatment in some form is necessary for borderline clients. The psychosocial skills training outlined in this manual is based on a model of treatment called dialectical behavior therapy (DBT). DBT is a broad-based cognitive–behavioral treatment developed specifically for BPD. It was the first psychotherapy shown via controlled clinical trials to be effective with this disorder (Linehan, Armstrong, Suarez, Allmon, & Heard, 1991; Linehan & Heard, 1993; Linehan, Heard, & Armstrong, in press). Psychosocial skills training is one portion of the treatment; the form of DBT that has been shown to be effective with borderline clients is a combination of individual psychotherapy and skills training.

DBT, including skills training, is based on a dialectical and biosocial theory of BPD. This chapter begins with a brief overview of the dialectical world view and the assumptions inherent in such a view. It then presents the biosocial theory of BPD and its development as well as the behavioral characteristics and dialectical dilemmas that are predicted from this theory.

Understanding the treatment philosophy and theoretical underpinnings of DBT as a whole is critical for effective use of this manual. The philosophy and theory are important because they determine therapists' attitude toward both treatment and their clients. This attitude, in turn, is an important component of therapists' relationship with their clients. The therapeutic relationship is central to effective treatment with suicidal and borderline individuals. This manual is a companion to my more complete text on DBT, *Cognitive–*

Behavioral Therapy for Borderline Personality Disorder, and these principles are discussed fully there. (Because I refer to that book very often throughout this manual, from here on I simply call it "the text.") The scientific underpinnings and references for many of my statements and positions are fully documented in Chapter 1 through 3 of the text; thus, I do not review or cite them here again.

World View and Basic Assumptions

As its name suggests, DBT is based on a dialectical world view. "Dialectics," as applied to behavior therapy, has two meanings: that of the fundamental nature of reality, and that of persuasive dialogue and relationship. As a world view or philosophical position, dialectics forms the basis of DBT. Alternatively, as dialogue and relationship, dialectics refers to the treatment approach or strategies used by the therapist to effect change. These strategies are described in full in Chapter 7 of the text and are summarized in Chapter 5 of this manual.

Dialectical perspectives on the nature of reality and human behavior share three primary characteristics, each of which is important in understanding BPD. First, much as dynamic systems perspectives do, dialectics stresses the fundamental interrelatedness or wholeness of reality. This means that a dialectical approach views analyses of individual parts of a system as of limited value per se unless the analysis clearly relates the part to the whole. Thus, dialectics directs our attention to the immediate and larger contexts of behavior, as well as to the interrelatedness of individual behavior patterns. With respect to skills training, a therapist must take into account first the interrelatedness of skills deficits. Learning one new set of skills is extremely difficult without learning other related skills simultaneously—a task that in itself is even more difficult. A dialectical view is also compatible with both contextual and feminist views of psychopathology. Learning psychosocial skills is particularly hard when a person's immediate environment or larger culture do not support such learning. Thus, the individual must learn not only self-regulation skills, but also better skills for influencing her environment. (Because the majority of borderline clients are women, and because the clinical trials demonstrating DBT's effectiveness were conducted with only women clients, I use the pronoun "she" and "her" throughout this manual to refer to a typical client. However, there is no reason to believe that the treatment would not be effective with men.)

Second, reality is not seen as static, but is comprised of internal opposing forces (thesis and antithesis) out of whose synthesis evolves a new set of opposing forces. A very important dialectical idea is that all propositions contain with them their own oppositions. As Goldberg (1980, pp. 295–296) put it, "I assume that truth is paradoxical, that each article of wisdom contains within it its own contradictions, that *truths stand side by side*" (emphasis Goldberg's). Dialectics, in this sense, is compatible with psychodynamic conflict models of psychopathology. Dichotomous and extreme thinking, behavior, and emotions, which are characteristic of BPD, are viewed as dialectical failures. The individual is stuck in polarities, unable to move to syntheses. With respect to psychosocial skills training, three of these polarities make progress extremely difficult. The therapist must pay attention to each and assist each client in moving toward a workable synthesis.

The first of these polarities is the dialectic between the need for the client to accept herself as she is in the moment and the need for her to change. This particular dialectic is the most fundamental tension in any psychotherapy, and it must be negotiated skillfully by the therapist if change is to occur. The second is the tension between the clients' getting what she needs and losing what she needs if she becomes more competent. I once had a client in skills training who every week reported doing none of the behavioral homework assignments and insisted that the treatment was not working. When after 6 months I suggested that maybe this wasn't the treatment for her, she reported that she had been trying the new skills all along and they *had* helped. However, she had not let me know about it because she was afraid that if she showed any improvement, I would dismiss her from skills training. A third very important polarity as to do with the client's maintaining personal integrity and validating her own views of her difficul-

ties versus learning new skills that will help her emerge from her suffering. If the client gets better by learning new skills, she validates her point that the problem all along was that she was unable to help herself. She has not been trying to manipulate people, as others have accused. She is not motivated to hurt others, or lacking in motivation altogether. But the client's learning new skills may also validate others' opinions: It may prove that they were right all along (and the client was wrong) —that the client was the problem, not the environment. Dialectics not only focuses the client's attention on these polarities, but also suggests ways out of them. (Ways out are discussed in Chapter 7 of the text.)

The third characteristic of dialectics is an assumption, following from the two above, that the fundamental nature of reality is change and process rather than content or structure. The most important implication here is that both the individual and the environment are undergoing continuous transition. Thus, therapy does not focus on maintaining a stable, consistent environment, but rather aims to help the client become comfortable with change. Within skills training itself, therapists must keep aware not only of how their clients are changing, but also of how both they themselves and the treatment they are applying are changing over time.

Biosocial Theory of Borderline Personality Disorder[2]

The main tenet of the biosocial theory is that the core disorder in BPD is emotion dysregulation. Emotion dysregulation is viewed as a joint outcome of biological disposition, environmental context, and the transaction between the two during development. The theory asserts that borderline individuals have difficulties in regulating several, if not all, emotions. This systemic dysregulation is produced by emotional vulnerability and by maladaptive and inadequate emotion modulation strategies.

Emotional vulnerability is defined by these characteristics: (1) very high sensitivity to emotional stimuli, (2) very intense response to emotional stimuli, and (3) a slow return to emotional baseline once emotional arousal has occurred. Emotion modulation is the ability to (1) inhibit inappropriate behavior related to strong negative or positive emotions, (2) organize oneself for coordinated action in the service of an external goal (i.e., act in a way that is not mood-dependent when necessary), (3) self-soothe any physiological arousal that the strong emotion has induced, and (4) refocus attention in the presence of strong emotion. Emotion dysregulation in borderline individuals then is the combination of an emotional response system that is oversensitive and overreactive with an inability to modulate the resulting strong emotions and actions associated with them. As a whole, the disposition to emotion dysregulation is biologically based (though not necessarily via heredity). A dysfunction in any part of the extremely complex human emotion regulation system can provide the biological basis for initial emotional vulnerability and subsequent difficulties in emotion modulation. Thus, the biological disposition may be different in different people, and it is not likely that we will ever find *one* biological abnormality that underlies all cases of BPD.

The Role of the Invalidating Environment in Emotion Dysregulation

The crucial developmental circumstance in producing the emotion dysregulation described above is the "invalidating environment." Such an environment is particularly damaging for the child who begins life with high emotional vulnerability. In turn, the emotionally vulnerable and reactive individual elicits invalidation from an environment that might have otherwise been supportive.

A defining characteristic of an invalidating environment is the tendency to respond erratically and inappropriately to private experience (e.g., beliefs, thoughts, feelings, sensations), and in particular to be insensitive to private experience that does not have public accompaniments. Invalidating environments also tend to respond in an extreme fashion (i.e., to overreact or underreact) to private experience that does have public accompaniments. Phenomenological, physiological, and cognitive components of emotions are prototypic private experiences that lead to invalidation in these settings. To clarify the invalidating environment's contribution to borderline behavioral patterns, let us contrast it to environments that foster more adaptive emotion regulation skills.

In the optimal family, public validation of private experience is given frequently. For example, when a child says she is thirsty, parents give her a drink (rather than saying, "No, you're not. You just had a drink"). When a child cries, parents soothe or attempt to find out what is wrong (rather than saying, "Stop being a crybaby!"). When a child expresses anger or frustration, family members take it seriously (rather than dismissing it as unimportant). When the child says, "I did my best," the parent agrees (rather than saying, "No, you didn't"). And so on. In the optimal family, the child's preferences (e.g., for color of room, activities, or clothes) are taken into account; the child's beliefs and thoughts are elicited and responded to seriously; and the child's emotions are viewed as important communications. Successful communication of private experience in such a family is followed by changes in other family members' behavior that increase the probability that the child's needs will be met and that decrease the probability of negative consequences. Parental responding that is attuned and nonaversive results in children who are better able to discriminate their own and others' emotions.

By contrast, an invalidating family is problematic because people in it respond to the communication of preferences, thoughts, and emotions nonattuned with responses—specifically, with either nonresponsiveness or more extreme consequences than more sensitive, validating social environments. This leads to an intensification of the differences between an emotionally vulnerable child's private experience and the experience the social environment actually supports and responds to. Persistent discrepancies between a child's private experience and what others in the environment describe or respond to as her experience provide the fundamental learning environment necessary for many of the behavioral problems associated with BPD.

In addition to early failures to respond optimally, an invalidating environment more generally emphasizes controlling emotional expressiveness, especially the expression of negative affect. Painful experiences are trivialized and attributed to negative traits such as lack of motivation, lack of discipline, and failure to adopt a positive attitude. Strong positive emotions and associated preferences may be attributed to traits such as lack of judgment and reflection or impulsivity. Other characteristics of the invalidating environment include restricting the demands a child may make upon the environment, discriminating against the child on the basis of gender or other arbitrary characteristics, and using punishment (from criticism up to physical and sexual abuse) to control behavior.

The invalidating environment contributes to emotion dysregulation by failing to teach the child to label and modulate arousal, to tolerate distress, or to trust her own emotional responses as valid interpretations of events. It also actively teaches the child to invalidate her own experiences by making it necessary for her to scan the environment for cues about how to act and feel, and by oversimplifying the ease of solving life's problems it fails to teach the child how to set realistic goals. Moreover, by punishing the expression of negative emotion and erratically reinforcing emotional communication only after escalation by the child, the family shapes an emotional expression style that vacillates between extreme inhibition and extreme disinhibition. In other words, the family's usual response to emotion cuts off the communicative function of ordinary emotions.

Emotional invalidation, particularly of negative emotions, is an interaction style characteristic of societies that put a premium on individualism, including individual self-control and individual achievement. Thus, it is quite characteristic of Western culture in general. A certain amount of invalidation is, of course, necessary in raising a child and teaching self-control. Not all communications of emotions, preferences, or beliefs can be responded to in a positive fashion. The child who is highly emotional and who has difficulty controlling emotional behaviors will elicit from the environment (especially parents, but also friends and teachers) the greatest efforts to control the emotionality from the outside. Invalidation can be quite effective at temporarily inhibiting emotional expression. Invalidating environments, however, have different effects on different children. The emotion control strategies used in invalidating families may have little negative impact on, or may even be useful to, some children who are physiologically well equipped to regulate their emotions. However, such strategies are hypothesized to have a devastating impact on emotionally vulnerable children. It is this interaction of biology and environment that is thought to result in BPD.

This transactional view of borderline development should not be used to diminish the importance of abusive environments in the etiology of BPD. One of the most traumatic invalidating experiences is childhood sexual abuse. Researchers have estimated that up to 75% of individuals with BPD have experienced some sort of sexual abuse in childhood. Histories of such abuse seem to distinguish borderline individuals from other outpatient diagnostic groups. This research strongly indicates childhood sexual abuse as an important factor in the development of BPD. It is unclear, however, whether the abuse in and of itself facilitates the development of borderline patterns, or whether the abuse and the development of the disorder both result from the extent of the familial dysfunction and invalidation. In other words, the history of victimization and the emotion regulation problems seen in borderline individuals may arise from the same set of developmental circumstances. Nevertheless, the high incidence of sexual abuse in individuals with BPD points to the possibility that this is a distinguishing precursor to the disorder.

The Pathogenesis of Emotion Dysregulation

Maccoby (1980) has argued that the inhibition of action is the basis for the organization of all behavior. The development of self-regulatory repertoires, especially the ability to inhibit and control affect, is one of the most important aspects of a child's development. The ability to regulate the experience and expression of emotion is crucial because its absence leads to the disruption of behavior, especially goal-directed behavior and other prosocial behavior. Alternatively, strong emotion re-

organizes or redirects behavior, preparing the individual for actions that compete with the nonemotionally or less emotionally driven behavioral repertoire.

The behavioral characteristics of borderline individuals can be conceptualized as the effects of emotion dysregualtion and maladaptive emotion regulation strategies. Impulsive behavior and especially parasuicide can be thought of as maladaptive but highly effective emotion regulation strategies. For example, overdosing usually leads to long periods of sleep, which in turn reduce susceptibility to emotion dysregulation. Although the mechanism by which self-mutilation exerts affect-regulating properties is not clear, it is very common for borderline individuals to report substantial relief from anxiety and other intense, negative emotional states following such acts. Suicidal behavior is also very effective in eliciting helping behaviors from the environment, which may be effective in avoiding or changing situations that elicit emotional pain. For example, suicidal behavior is generally the most effective way for a nonpsychotic individual to be admitted to an inpatient psychiatric unit. Finally, engaging in a parasuicidal act (and its aftereffects if it becomes public) can reduce painful emotions by providing a compelling distraction.

The inability to regulate emotional arousal also interferes with the development and maintenance of a sense of self. Generally, one's sense of self is formed by observations of oneself and of others' reactions to one's actions. Emotional consistency and predictability, across time and similar situations, are prerequisites of identity development. Unpredictable emotional lability leads to unpredictable behavior and cognitive inconsistency, and consequently interferes with identity development. The tendency of borderline individuals to inhibit or attempt to inhibit emotional responses may also contribute to an absence of a strong sense of identity. The numbness associated with inhibited affect is often experienced as emptiness, further contributing to an inadequate and at times completely absent sense of self. Similarly, if an individual's sense of events is never "correct" or is unpredictably "correct"—the situation in an invalidating environment—then the individual may be expected to develop an overdependence on others.

Effective interpersonal relationships depend on both a stable sense of self and a capacity for spontaneity in emotional expression. Successful relationships also require a capacity to self-regulate emotions in appropriate ways and to tolerate some emotionally painful stimuli. Emotion regulation difficulties interfere with a stable sense of self and with normal emotional expression. Without such capabilities, it is understandable that borderline individuals develop chaotic relationships. These individuals' difficulties in controlling impulsive behaviors and expressions of extreme negative emotions wreak havoc in many ways with their relationships; in particular, difficulties with anger and anger expression preclude the maintenance of stable relationships.

The Treatment Program

DBT applies a broad array of cognitive and behavior therapy strategies to the problem of BPD, including suicidal behaviors. Like standard cognitive–behavioral therapy programs, DBT emphasizes ongoing assessment and data collection on current behaviors; clear and precise definition of treatment targets; and a collaborative working relationship between therapist and client, including attention to orienting the client to the therapy program and mutual commitment to treatment goals. Many components of DBT—problem solving, exposure, skills training, contingency management, and cognitive modification—have been prominent in cognitive and behavior therapies for years.

Stylistically, DBT blends a matter-of-fact, somewhat irreverent, and at times outrageous attitude about current and previous parasuicidal and other dysfunctional behaviors with therapist warmth, flexibility, responsiveness to the client, and strategic self-disclosure. The continuing efforts in DBT to "reframe" suicidal and other dysfunctional behaviors as part of the client's learned problem-solving repertoire, and to focus therapy on active problem solving, are balanced by a corresponding emphasis on validating the client's current emotional, cognitive, and behavioral responses just as they are. The problem-solving focus requires that the therapist address all problematic client behaviors (in and out of sessions) and therapy situations in a systematic manner, including conducting a collaborative behavioral analysis, formulating hypotheses about possible variables influencing the problem, generating possible changes (behavioral solutions), and trying out and evaluating the solutions.

The attention to contingencies operating within the therapeutic environment requires the therapist to pay close attention to the reciprocal influence that therapist and client have on each other. Although natural contingencies are highlighted as a means of influencing client behavior, the therapist is not prohibited from using arbitrary reinforcers as well as aversive contingencies when the behavior in question is lethal or the behavior required of the client is not readily produced under ordinary therapeutic conditions. The tendency of borderline individuals to actively avoid threatening situations is a continuing focus of DBT. Both in-session and *in vivo* exposures to fear-eliciting stimuli are arranged and encouraged. The emphasis on cognitive modification is less systematic than in pure cognitive therapy, but none-the-less it is

viewed as an important component both in ongoing behavioral analysis and in promoting change.

The focus on validating the client's thoughts, feelings, and actions requires that the DBT therapist search for the grain of wisdom or truth inherent in each client response and communicate that wisdom to the client. A belief in the client's essential desire to grow and progress, as well as a belief in her inherent capability to change, underpins the treatment. Validation also involves frequent sympathetic acknowledgment of the client's sense of emotional desperation. The whole of treatment emphasizes building and maintaining a positive, interpersonal, collaborative relationship between client and therapist. A major characteristic of the therapeutic relationship is that the primary role of the therapist is as consultant to the client, *not* consultant to other individuals. The therapist is consistently on the side of the client.

Modifications of Cognitive and Behavior Therapies for Borderline Individuals

Standard cognitive and behavior therapies were originally developed for individuals without serious personality disorders. Over the years, however, they have been applied increasingly to individuals who also have personality disorders, including BPD. The applications of cognitive–behavioral therapy to individuals with BPD has required some changes of emphasis and expansion of theoretical underpinnings. In DBT four areas are emphasized that, while not new, have not received as much attention in traditional cognitive–behavioral applications: (1) the emphasis on acceptance and validation of behavior as it is in the moment; (2) the emphasis on treating therapy-interfering behaviors of both client and therapist; (3) the emphasis on the therapeutic relationship as essential to the treatment; and (4) the emphasis on dialectic processes. First, DBT emphasizes acceptance of current behavior and reality more so than most cognitive and behavior therapies. To a great extent, in fact, standard cognitive–behavioral therapy can be thought of as a technology of change. It derives many of its techniques from the field of learning, which is the study of behavioral change through experience. In contrast, DBT emphasizes the importance of balancing the technology of change and a technology of acceptance. Although acceptance of clients as they are is crucial to any good therapy, DBT goes a step further than standard cognitive–behavioral therapy in emphasizing the necessity of teaching clients to fully accept themselves and their world as they are in the moment. The acceptance advocated is quite radical—it is not acceptance in order to create change. The focus on acceptance in DBT is an integration of Eastern psychological and spiritual practices (primarily Zen practice) in Western approaches to treatment.

The emphasis in DBT on therapy-interfering behaviors is more similar to the psychodynamic emphasis on "transference" behaviors and "countertransference" behaviors than to anything in standard cognitive–behavioral therapies. Generally behavior therapists have given little empirical attention to the treatment of client behaviors that interfere with the treatment. (The exceptions here are the large literature on treatment compliance behaviors, and the various approaches generally described under the rubric of "shaping"; the latter have received a fair amount of attention in the treatment of children, chronic psychiatric inpatients, and the mentally retarded.) This is not to say that the problem has been ignored completely. Patterson and his colleagues have even developed a measure of treatment resistance for use with families undergoing his behavioral family interventions (Chamberlain, Patterson, Reid, Kavanagh, & Forgatch, 1984; Patterson & Forgatch, 1985). Although the situation is beginning to change, almost no attention to date has been given to understanding therapist behaviors that interfere with effective cognitive–behavioral treatments.

My emphasis on the therapeutic relationship as crucial to therapeutic progress in DBT comes primarily from my work in interventions with suicidal individuals. At times, it is only the relationship that keeps such a person alive. In psychosocial skills training, the relationship between client and therapist (and, in group settings, the relationship among clients) is also a powerful force in keeping the patient in the therapy. Borderline individuals are notorious for dropping out of therapy early; thus, attention must be paid to factors that will enhance their attachment both to therapy and to life itself. Finally, the focus on dialectical processes sets DBT off from standard cognitive–behavioral therapy, but not as much as it appears at first glance. For example, contextual theories are very close to dialectical thinking. The emphasis in cognitive therapy on the interrelationships within the person between different types of behavior (e.g., the influence of cognitive behavior on emotional behavior) is also compatible with a dialectical perspective.

Whether these differences between DBT and standard cognitive and behavior therapies are fundamentally important is, of course, an empirical question. Certainly, when all is said and done, the standard cognitive–behavioral components may be the ones primarily responsible for the effectiveness of DBT. Or, as cognitive and behavior therapies expand their scope, we may find that the differences between them and DBT are not as sharp as I suggest.

Relationship Between Individual Psychotherapy and Skills Training

DBT was developed from a model of BPD as a combination of motivation problems and capability deficits. First, according to the argument laid down above, borderline individuals lack important self-regulation, interpersonal, and distress tolerance skills. In particular, they are unable either to inhibit maladaptive mood-dependent behaviors or to initiate behaviors that are independent of current mood and necessary to meet long-range goals. Second, strong emotions and associated dysfunctional assumptions and beliefs learned in the original invalidating environment, together with continuing invalidating environments, form a motivational context that inhibits the use of behavioral skills the person does have and often reinforces inappropriate borderline behaviors. As my colleagues and I developed this treatment approach, however, it quickly became apparent that (1) psychosocial skills training to the extent we believe necessary is extraordinarily difficult if not impossible within the context of a therapy oriented to reducing the motivation to die and/or act in a borderline fashion; and (2) sufficient attention to motivational issues cannot be given in a treatment with the rigorous control of therapy agenda needed for skills training. From this was born the idea of splitting the therapy into two components: one that focuses primarily on psychosocial skills training and one that focuses primarily on motivational issues, including the motivation to stay alive, to replace borderline behaviors with skillful behavior, and to build a life worth living.

Relationship of Borderline Behavioral Patterns to Skills Training

The criteria for BPD as currently defined (see Chapter 1 of the text for a detailed discussion) reflect a pattern of behavioral, emotional, and cognitive instability and dysregulation. These difficulties can be summarized into five categories; in DBT four specific skills training modules are aimed directly at these five categories. First, as I have been discussing, borderline individuals generally experience dysregulation and lability of emotions. Emotional responses are reactive, and the individuals generally have problems with anger and anger expression as well as with episodic depression, anxiety, and irritability. One DBT skills training module aims to teach emotion regulation skills.

Second, borderline individuals often experience interpersonal dysregulation. Their relationships are usually chaotic, intense, and marked with difficulties. Despite this, borderline individuals often find it extremely hard to let go of relationships; instead, they may engage in intense and frantic efforts to keep significant individuals from leaving them. More so than most, borderline individuals seem to do well when in stable, positive relationships and to do poorly when not in stable relationships. Thus, another DBT skills training module aims to teach interpersonal effectiveness skills.

Third, borderline individuals have patterns of behavioral dysregulation, as evidenced by extreme and problematic impulsive behaviors as well as by attempts to injure, mutilate, or kill themselves. Impulsive and suicidal behaviors are viewed in DBT as maladaptive problem-solving behaviors resulting from an individual's inability to tolerate emotional distress long enough to pursue potentially more effective solutions. Therefore, one DBT skills training module aims to teach distress tolerance skills.

Fourth, dysregulation of the sense of self is common. It is not unusual for a borderline individual to report having no sense of a self at all, feeling empty, and not knowing who she is. And fifth, brief, nonpsychotic cognitive disturbances (including depersonalization, dissociation, and delusions) are at times brought on by stressful situations and usually clear up when the stress is ameliorated. To address both types of dysregulation, one DBT skills training module aims to teach a core set of "mindfulness" skills—that is, skills having to do with the ability to consciously experience and observe oneself and surrounding events.

A Look Ahead

In the next four chapters I discuss practical aspects of skills training; session format and starting skills training; the applications of DBT structural strategies and skills training procedures to formal skills training; and the application of other DBT strategies and procedures to skills training. Together, these chapters set the stage for deciding how to conduct skills training in a particular clinic or practice. The following five chapters offer specific guidelines on how to teach the behavioral skills that together make up the formal skills training component of DBT. I should note here that although we do conduct individual skills training in my clinic, all such training in our clinical trials were conducted in groups. Many of the treatment guidelines in this manual assume that skills training is being conducted in groups, mainly because it is easier to adapt group skills training techniques to work with individual clients than vice versa. (The issue of group versus individual skills training is discussed at some length in the next chapter.)

Notes

1. Psychotherapists usually use either the word "patient' or the word "client" to refer to an individual receiving psychotherapy. In this manual, I use the term "client" consistently; in the companion text, I use the term "patient." A reasonable case can be made for using either term. The case for using the term "client" can be found in the definition of the term given by the *Original Oxford English Dictionary on Compact Disc 1987*: "A person who employs the services of a professional or business man or woman in any branch of business, or for whom the latter acts in a professional capacity; a customer." The emphasis here is on the professional nature of the relationship and services offered (skills training), rather than on the presumed "illness" of the person receiving services. Other, less common uses of the term—such a "One who is under the protection or patronage of another, a dependent" (as in "client state"), or "An adherent or follower of a master"—are less applicable, as they do not fully convey the independent status accorded the client in DBT skills training.

2. The ideas in this section are drawn not only from the text but from Linehan and Koerner (1992), which is a condensed discussion of the biosocial theory of BPD.

2

Practical Issues in Psychosocial Skills Training

Psychosocial skills training is necessary when solutions to an individual's problems and attainment of her desired goals require behavioral skills not currently in her behavioral repertoire. That is, under ideal circumstances (where behavior is not interfered with by fears, conflicting motives, unrealistic beliefs, etc.), the individual cannot generate or produce the behaviors required. The term "skills" in DBT is used synonymously with "ability," and includes in its broadest sense cognitive, emotional, and overt behavioral (or action) skills together with their integration, which is necessary for effective performance. Effectiveness is gauged by both direct and indirect effects of the behavior. Effective performance can be defined as those behaviors that lead to a maximum of positive outcomes with a minimum of negative outcomes. Thus, "skills" is used in the sense of "using skillful means," as well as in the sense of responding to situations adaptively or effectively.

The emphasis on integration of behaviors to produce a skillful response is important. Very often (indeed, usually), an individual has the component behaviors of a skills but cannot put them together coherently when necessary. For example, an interpersonally skillful response requires putting together words the person already knows into effective sentences, together with appropriate body language, intonation, eye contact, and so forth. The parts are rarely new; the combination, however, often is. In the terminology of DBT, almost any desired behavior can be thought of as a skill. Thus, coping actively and effectively with problems and avoiding maladaptive or ineffective responses are both considered using one's skills. The central aim of DBT as a whole is to replace ineffective, maladaptive, or nonskilled behavior with skillful responses. The aim of DBT skills

training is to help the individual acquire the needed skills.

Individual versus Group Skills Training

Successful psychosocial skills training requires discipline by both client and therapist. In skills training, the therapy agenda is set by the skills to be learned. In typical psychotherapy and in DBT individual psychotherapy, by contrast, the agenda is usually set by the current problems of the client. When current problems are pressing, staying with a skills training agenda requires the therapist to take a very active role, controlling the direction and focus of the session. Most therapists are not trained to take such a directive role; and thus, despite their good intentions, their efforts at skills training often peter out as clients' problems escalate.

Even therapists who are well trained in directive treatment strategies have great difficulty keeping to a directive agenda when treating borderline clients. The inevitable crises and low emotional pain tolerance of such clients constitute a major and continuing problem. It is difficult for the clients, and consequently for their therapists, to attend to anything but the current crises during treatment sessions. For some clients even daily sessions would not solve the problem, since they often seem to be in an unrelenting state of crisis. It is particularly difficult to stay focused on skills when a client threatens to commit suicide if her current pain is not taken seriously. Taking it seriously usually means forgoing the day's skills training agenda in favor of resolving the current crisis.

Other clients may be less demanding of therapist

time and energy, but their passivity, hopelessness, and/or lack of interest in skills training may pose a formidable roadblock. It is easy in such a case for the therapist to get worn out with the client and just give up the effort, especially if the therapist is not a firm believer in skills training anyway. Skills training can also be relatively boring for therapists, especially for those who have done considerable skills training with other clients. It is like doing the same operation over and over and over. Clients' fluctuating moods from week to week and within the therapy session (a characteristic of borderline individuals), together with therapists' wavering interest, can create havoc with the best-laid skills training plans.

Inadequate attention to the actual teaching of behavioral skills, and the resulting therapy drift, are particularly likely in individual as opposed to group skills training. First, in individual therapy there is often nothing outside of the two participants to keep therapy on track. If both client and therapist want to switch to something else, they can do it easily. By contrast, in group therapy other clients — or at least therapists' sense of obligation to other clients — keeps therapists on track, even when one client wants to change track. Second, when one client in group skills training is not in the mood for learning skills, others may be. The reinforcement these other clients give the therapist for continuing skills training can be more powerful than the punishment delivered by the client who is not in the mood.

The crux of the problem is this: Skills training with a borderline individual is often not immediately reinforcing for either her or her therapist. There is rarely a sense of immediate relief. Nor is psychosocial skills training as interesting as having "heart-to-hearts," a topic I have discussed in Chapter 12 of the text. Skills training requires much more active work for both client and therapist. Thus, for individual skills training to work, special precautions must be made for arranging events so that *both* therapist and client will find it reinforcing enough to continue.

Much of the development of DBT was influenced by the dual task of finding a treatment that would be effective in helping borderline individuals and a treatment that therapists could actually apply on a day-to-day basis. As I have noted in Chapter 1 of this manual, the difficulties of conducting skills training within the context of individual psychotherapy led me to split the treatment into components, with the acquisition of skills as the goal of one treatment component and getting the client to use the skills in place of maladaptive behaviors as the goal of another component (i.e., individual psychotherapy). Put in the vernacular, skills training tries to cram the skills into the person and individual psychotherapy tries to pull them out.

For the reasons discussed above, the standard mode of skills training in DBT is group therapy. A number of circumstances, however, may make it preferable or necessary to conduct skills training with an individual client rather than in a group. In a private practice setting or a small clinic, there may not be more than one client needing skills training at any one time, or a therapist may not be able to organize more than one person at a time for skills training. Some clients are not appropriate for groups. Although in my experience this is very rare, a client who cannot inhibit overt hostile behavior toward other group members should not be put into a group until this behavior is under control. Some clients may have already participated in 1 or more years of a skills training group but need further focused attention to one category or set of skills. Finally, a client may not be able to attend the offered group sessions.

Individual Skills Training

Again, focused skills training on an individual basis with a borderline client requires enormous self-discipline and perseverance on the part of the therapist. On the client's side, the major roadblocks are her attempts to divert a skills training session to other, more pressing topics, or her refusal or inability to participate in skills training the therapist is attempting to provide. On the therapist's side, the major roadblocks are discomfort with active, directive interventions, or the therapist's lack of interest, boredom, or inability to provide the skills guidance that the client is begging for. Treatment in these cases can easily become a power struggle between the client and therapist. If the therapist of the client who disrupts skills training can hold out, and maintain his or her focus on the client's long-term needs over the short term needs, I think that individual skills training can work. Such a focus, however, is very difficult to maintain in the face of what are often genuine life crises. As for the therapist roadblocks, the intent of this manual is to generate some interest (and even some enthusiasm) in the therapist who is uninterested, and to provide guidelines and advice for the therapist who feels unable to offer skills training. Even for an interested skillful therapist, however, skills training with borderline clients is difficult. As I have noted in the text, trying to conduct skills training with a borderline individual is like trying to teach a person how to put up a tent in the middle of a hurricane.

Nonetheless, it is also the case that if the client had more effective skills in her repertoire, she would be able to cope much better with crisis situations. And this is the dilemma: How does the therapist teach the skills necessary to cope, when the client's current inability to cope is so great that she is not receptive to acquiring new behavioral responses? One solution is for the therapist simply to make continuous efforts to incorporate the skills training procedures in every session. A problem with this approach is that it is often not apparent to the client in individual therapy what contingencies are operating at any given time in a session; the rules are not clear. The client who wants to focus on an immediate solution to an immediate crisis, therefore, has no guidelines as to when insisting on such attention is appropriate and likely to be reinforced and when it is not. A problem for the therapist is that it is extremely difficult to remain on track. My own inability to do just this was one of the important factors in the development of DBT as it is today.

A second alternative is to have a second therapist or behavioral technician do individual skills training with each client. The rules for client and therapist behavior in this case are clear. In this format, general behavioral skills are learned with the skills trainer; crises, including the application of skills learned to particular crisis situations, are the focus of individual psychotherapy. This approach seems especially advantageous in certain situations. For example, in our university clinic a number of students are eager to obtain experience in working with individuals who meet criteria for BPD but are not able to commit to longer-term individual therapy. Conducting focused skills training is a good opportunity for these students, and, in my experience, has worked out well for the clients. It would be as easy in any setting where psychiatric residents, social workers or psychiatric nurses are in training. In a group clinical practice, therapists may conduct skills training for each other; a large practice may hire some therapists with specific talents in this area. The treatment model here is somewhat similar to a general practitioner's sending a client to a specialist for specialized treatment. The difference in DBT is that routine (possibly weekly) meetings between individual psychotherapists and skills trainers are probably essential to the success of psychosocial skills training for borderline clients. I discuss this point further below.

An individual therapist who has no one to refer a client to for skills training, or who wants to do it himself or herself, should make the context of skills training different from that of usual psychotherapy. For example, a separate weekly meeting devoted specifically to skills training may be scheduled. If possible, the session should be conducted in a room different from that used for individual psychotherapy. Other possibilities include switching chairs; moving a table or desk near (or between) the therapist and the client to put your skills training materials on; using a blackboard; turning up the lighting; having skills training sessions at a different time of day than psychotherapy sessions, or for a shorter or longer time period; arranging to audiotape or videotape the sessions if this is not done in individual psychotherapy, or vice versa; and billing differently. For

a therapist with a particularly difficult client, participation in a supervision/consultation group is important in keeping up motivation and focusing on skills.

Group Skills Training

I have already mentioned a number of disadvantages to individual skills training. The chief disadvantage not yet mentioned is that it is inefficient. Even though in our experience borderline clients almost never want to join a group at the beginning, group treatment has much to offer over and above what any individual therapy can offer. First, therapists have an opportunity to observe and work with interpersonal behaviors that show up in peer relationships but may only rarely occur in individual therapy sessions. Second, clients have an opportunity to interact with other people like themselves, and the resulting validation and development of a support group are, in my opinion, very therapeutic. Third, clients have an opportunity to learn from one another thus increasing avenues of therapeutic input. Fourth, groups typically reduce the intensity of the personal relationship between individual clients and the group psychotherapist; in dynamic terms, the transference is diluted. This can be very important, because the intensity of therapy sometimes creates more problems than it solves for borderline clients. Finally, skills groups offer a relatively non-threatening opportunity for individual clients to learn how to be in a group. This can be very important for two reasons. First, people in general, as well as borderline individuals, have to be able to function well in groups. Second, in our treatment program further supportive process groups are offered. These groups not only are very therapeutic when combined with individual psychotherapy, but also offer a long-term treatment that may be more dependable and economical than long-term individual therapy.

In my psychotherapy research program, all clients in individual therapy also participate in group skills training. This requirement is made clear to each client at the initial screening meeting. In my own clinical practice, I may refuse to work individually with clients who are unwilling to participate in group skills training if I believe that their skills deficits are such that individual psychotherapy will be severely hampered without the addition of skills training. Indeed, one of the reasons (among many others) for the focus in DBT on building a strong, positive interpersonal relationship with a client in individual therapy is that the therapist will be able to persuade her to participate in group skills training even when she very much does not want to. In our research program, initial resistance to group skills training has been more the rule than the exception.

A group can include as few as two people. In our

clinic, with very dysfunctional clients, we try to have six to eight persons in each group. A number of issues are particularly important in group therapy; I discuss many of these throughout the book. (You can, of course, simply ignore them if you are conducting individual skills training.)

Open versus Closed Groups

In open groups, new members can enter on a continuing basis. In closed groups, a group is formed and stays together for a certain time period; new members are not allowed once the group composition is stable. Whether a group is open or closed will often depend on pragmatic issues. In many clinical settings, especially inpatient units, open groups are a necessity. In outpatient settings, however, it may be possible to round up a number of people who want skills training and who will agree to stay together for a period of time. If a choice is available, which type of group works better?

I have tried both types of groups and believe that open groups work better for skills training, although closed groups may work as well or better for subsequent supportive process therapy groups. Why? There are two reasons. First, in an open group clients have an opportunity to learn to cope with change in a relatively stable environment. Borderline individuals often have enormous difficulty with change; they may also have difficulties with trust. They may implore the therapists to keep the group stable and unchanging. However, keeping the group open, with somewhat controlled but continual change, allows therapeutic exposure to change in a context where clients can be helped to respond to it effectively. I once asked a client how she felt about new members' occasionally entering an open group and older members' leaving. She responded that she figured I had arranged it that way so she could practice her distress tolerance skills. After running a closed group for a year, where we tried to provide constancy and stability, I was shocked to learn that we could not make even minor changes in starting a second year without intense resistance on the part of group members. For example, we tried to move the table around which members sat, and ended up in a 3-week power struggle (until I gave in and agreed to keep the table).

Second, in a closed group it becomes progressively easier to deviate from the skills training agenda. Process issues frequently become more prominent as members get more comfortable with one another. The group as a whole can begin to drift away from a rigorous focus on learning behavioral skills. Although process issues are obviously important and cannot be ignored, there is a definite difference between a behavioral skills train-

ing group and an interpersonal process group. The supportive process groups in DBT follow the skills groups; they are not offered until after an individual has gone through all of the skills training. Periodically adding new skills training group members, who expect to learn new behavioral skills, forces the group to get back on task.

Treatment Module Cycles

Four skills training modules have been developed for DBT: (1) core mindfulness skills, (2) interpersonal effectiveness skills, (3) emotion regulation skills, and (4) distress tolerance skills. The rationale for focusing on these particular skills has been discussed briefly in Chapter 1 of this manual and more extensively in Chapter 5 of the text. General group format and therapy strategies and procedures, as well as specific content for each module, are presented in later chapters.

The interpersonal effectiveness, emotion regulation, and distress tolerance modules can be covered in 8 weeks (if training stays focused). Core mindfulness skills can be covered in two to three sessions, and then are reviewed and expanded upon further at the beginning of each of the other modules. Clients in my clinic generally stay in psychosocial skills training for at least 1 year. This means that each client goes through each eight week module twice. Because mindfulness skills are reviewed at the beginning of each module and are woven through each of the other three modules, the skills taught here are covered many times over the year. Some clients in our clinic have participated for more than 1 year, although usually clients "graduate" to more advanced groups after going through each module twice. A well-functioning client might profitably graduate from skills training after 6 months.

A number of psychiatric inpatient units are presently using DBT. One long-term psychiatric hospital accepts clients for a 6-month structured treatment program. Clients go through each skills module once; they can also review the videotaped sessions as often as they wish. The modules can then be repeated as necessary in outpatient therapy. Day treatment settings may offer several modules concurrently, with clients attending more than one at a time. Short-term, acute inpatient units, may offer just one or two of the modules. For example, a number of such units offer a package combining mindfulness and distress tolerance skills. Other units have taken a few skills from each module and constructed a shortened version of DBT skills training. As these examples indicate, the treatment modules lend themselves to mixing and matching to suit particular needs and treatment philosophies. All other things being equal, however, I would suggest teaching straight from the manual a few times before beginning to change and modify the skills treatment.

Massed versus Spaced Practice

Although each training module is designed to take 8 weeks to cover, up to a year could be spent on each. The content for each skills area is comprehensive and complex for such a short period of time. Covering the skills training material in this brief number of weeks requires very strict time management. Therapists also have to be willing to go on even when some (or even all) clients have not acquired the skills that are currently being taught. Clients are often overwhelmed with the amount of information the first time they go through each module. So why not expand each module to one 16-week module (massed practice) rather than two 8-week modules (spaced practice)? There are several reasons for the present format.

First, borderline individuals are variable in their mood and functionality. They often go through periods of several weeks where they may miss meetings or, when present, pay attention minimally (if at all). Presenting material twice increases the probability that each person will be present, both physically and psychologically, at least once when a particular segment is covered.

Second, different clients have different needs; thus, the modules are differentially relevant and preferred by various individuals. Having to sit though a disliked module for 16 weeks is very difficult. Sitting though 8 weeks of a disliked module is also hard, but not as hard.

Third, in a 16-week format, the modules scheduled second and third get less practice time than in an 8-week format. If I could make a case that one module is indeed the most important and needs the most practice, this would not be a liability. However, I have no controlled empirical data to use in choosing which module that would be. In addition, it is doubtful that one module would be best for all clients. The central premise of a skills-oriented behavioral therapy is that acquisition of behavioral skills requires extensive practice. Even though the material often feels overwhelming the first time when presented in the 8-week format, clients nonetheless seem able to practice the skills in their everyday lives. Thus, presenting each module once during the first 6 months of treatment leaves a minimum of 6 months for continued practice before skill training ends.

Fourth, going over the material after having had a chance to practice the skills for several months can be beneficial. The material makes more sense. And it offers the chance for the clients to learn that problems that seem really hard at one point may not always seem so hard if they persevere in their attempts to overcome them.

Finally, my experience has been that when 16 weeks are allotted to cover a treatment module, it is far easier to divert therapy time to attending to individual clients' crises and process issues. Although some attention must be given to these issues, it is easy to drift out of skills training and toward supportive process therapy, when time is not of the essence. In my experience, once this has happened, it is extremely difficult to get back control of the therapy agenda.

Even though I see several advantages for the 8-week format, there is no *a priori* reason for it. And moving so quickly through each module depends on very close coordination with each client's individual therapist (when this person is not a skills trainer). Again, in DBT it is the task of the individual psychotherapy to help the client use the new behaviors she is learning in the everyday situations where they are needed, including crises. The individual psychotherapy is also charged with analyzing motivational problems that interfere with replacing maladaptive behaviors with the DBT behavioral skills.

Ordering of Modules

At this writing, there are no empirical data to suggest how to order the modules. Since the core mindfulness skills are woven throughout each of the three training modules, mindfulness obviously has to be the first module presented. In our current program, the interpersonal effectiveness, emotion regulation, and distress tolerance modules follow, in that order. The rationale for this is based on the increasing abstractness of the skills and principles over the three modules. In addition, the three modules in this order can be viewed as decreasing in their degree of validation of a client's sense of emotional pain.

The interpersonal effectiveness module is presented as teaching skills in changing pain-producing environments. The situation is so pain-producing that it has to be changed. The emotion regulation module assumes that even though the situation may be generating pain, the individual's response is so painful that it also has to change, and can be changed. The distress tolerance module assumes that even though there may be a lot of pain, it can be tolerated, and life can be accepted and lived in spite of pain. Surely, this is a difficult lesson for anyone, especially for our clients. One can, however, make a reasonably good case for any order of modules. In my own clinic now (some other centers do the same), we give clients the "Crisis Survival Strategies" handout (part of the distress tolerance module) during the first meeting with the client. These skills are more or less self-explanatory, and many clients find them extremely helpful. We then go over them in detail when we teach the distress tolerance module.

Heterogeneous versus Homogeneous Groups

DBT skills training group members in my clinic are homogeneous with respect to diagnosis: they are restricted to individuals who meet criteria for BPD and who have engaged in recent parasuicidal acts (intentional self-injurious behaviors; see Chapter 1 of the text for a full explanation of this term). Group members are not particularly homogeneous in other ways. Ages range from 16 to 48 years; some groups include clients of both sexes; and socioeconomic, marital, and parental statuses vary. For all of our clients so far, our group has represented their first experience of being with other individuals sharing very similar difficulties. Although from my perspective a homogeneous group is an asset in doing group therapy with this population, the choice obviously has its pros and cons.

Arguments Against a Homogeneous Group

There are a number of rather strong arguments against a homogeneous group of suicidal, borderline clients. First, such a group is risky on an outpatient basis. Any kind of therapy, individual or group, can be very stressful for borderline clients. Their extreme emotional reactivity all but insures that intense emotions will be aroused, requiring skillful therapeutic management. A therapist has to be very good at reading and responding to nonverbal cues and indirect verbal communications—a difficult task under the best of circumstances. Therapeutic comments are often misinterpreted, or interpreted in a way that the therapist did not mean and insensitive comments have a strong impact. With even the most vigilant and sensitive therapist, there will often be times when a client leaves an individual therapy session in more emotional turmoil than when she came in. Frequent phone calls are often needed to resolve the issue.

These problems are simply compounded in group therapy. It is impossible for one or two therapists to track and respond individually to each group member's emotional responses to a therapy session. With more clients and a faster pace than in individual therapy, there are more opportunities for therapists to make mistakes and insensitive remarks, as well as for clients to misconstrue what is going on. In addition, it is more difficult for a client to express her emotional reactions to a group therapist in front of other group members. Thus the possibility for clients leaving in turmoil, with emotional responses they cannot handle, is greatly increased in group over individual therapy.

A second, related drawback to homogeneous groups has to do with the tendency of clients to become emotionally involved with one anothers' problems and tragedies. Clients often become anxious, angry, depressed, and hopeless not only about the problems in their own lives, but also about the problems of those close to them. Thus, just listening to others' life descriptions can precipitate intense, painful emotional responses. This problem has been a very difficult issue for us staff members to handle among ourselves; we also have to listen to painful story after story from our clients. Imagine how much more difficult it is for individuals who have little capacity to modulate their responses to emotionally charged information.

Another argument against homogeneous groups is based on the notion that in a group with only borderline clients, there will be no one to model appropriate, adaptive behaviors—or, similarly, that there will be extensive modeling of inappropriate behaviors. I have simply not found this to be the case. In fact, I am frequently amazed at the capacity of our clients to be helpful to one another in coping with life's problems. The one area where an absence of appropriate modeling does seem to exist is in the area of coping with extreme negative feelings. Especially at the beginning of treatment, it is often necessary for the group leaders to take much of the responsibility for modeling how to cope with negative emotions in a nonsuicidal manner.

A fourth argument against homogeneous groups has to do with the active passivity of borderline individuals (see Chapter 3 of the text for a description of this behavioral pattern), their ability to "catch" others' moods and behavior, and their inability to act in a mood-independent fashion. Contagion of suicidal behavior can be a particularly difficult problem. At times, if one group member comes to a session in a discouraged or depressed mood, all members of the group will soon be feeling the same way. If group leaders are not careful, even they can sink down with the members. One of the reasons why we have two leaders for each group in our clinic (for further discussion, see below) is that when this happens, each therapist will have someone to keep him or her functioning at an energetic level. It can be very difficult.

Finally, it is sometimes said that the borderline clients are more prone to "attention seeking" than are other clients, and that this tendency will be disruptive to any group process. Once again, I have not found this to be the case.

Arguments for a Homogeneous Group

From my perspective, there are two powerful arguments for a homogeneous group. First, homogeneity allows the group leaders to tailor the skills and theoretical conceptions offered specifically for problems of suicidal behaviors and BPD. Most of the skills taught are applicable for many client populations. However, a heterogeneous group would require a much more generic presentation of the skills, and the application of the skills to each person's central problems would have to be worked out individually. A common conceptual scheme would be difficult to present unless it was very general.

A second argument for a homogeneous group is the opportunity for clients to be with a group of individuals who share the same problems and concerns. In my experience, this is a very powerful validating experience for our clients. Many have been in other groups. As noted above, however, they have not had the experience of being around others who actually understand the often inexplicable urges to injure themselves, the desire to be dead, the frustration of being unable to control emotions and behavior, and the pain of emotional invalidating experiences. All know intimately the difficulty of confronting emotional pain in anything other than a maladaptive way.

A factor that can complicate the advantage of having an entire group of suicidal individuals has to do with different rates of individual progress in treatment. When one client is engaging in frequent self-injury and suicide attempts, it is very validating to have other group members struggling with the same issue. However, once the client has stopped such behaviors, it can be very hard for herself if others are still engaging in the self-injurious behaviors. Hearing about others' self-injury and overdoses seems to cause a greater urge to do the same thing; this is, of course, a threatening experience for the person who is working hard at avoiding self-harm. In addition, we have found that as a client progresses in therapy, she often begins to change her self-image from that of "borderline person" to that of "nonborderline person." Especially if she is still judgmental, she can find it very hard to stay in a group defined as a group for borderline individuals. These two issues—the urge to imitate suicidal behavior, and the need to change one's self-image from borderline to nonborderline—must be dealt with effectively by the group leaders if an individual is to continue with the group.

The Role of Individual Psychotherapy in Psychosocial Skills Training

As I have said previously, skills training with suicidal, borderline clients is an adjunct to individual psychotherapy. It is a part of DBT; it is not the total treatment. The key idea in DBT skills training is that it is the servant of individual psychotherapy, so to speak. It provides the clay that the individual therapist and client can use together to mold a functional figure. With severely dys-

functional borderline clients skills training cannot stand alone. This point is crucial to keep in mind.

What kind of individual psychotherapy works best with skills training? Our research data suggest that DBT individual therapy plus DBT skills training is superior to non-DBT individual therapy plus skills training (Linehan, Heard, & Armstrong, 1993). Therapists conducting skills training, however, may not always have control over the type of individual psychotherapy their clients get. This is especially likely in community mental health settings and inpatient psychiatric units. In settings where DBT is just being introduced, there simply may not be enough DBT individual therapists to go around. Or a unit may be trying to integrate different approaches to treatment. For example, a number of psychiatric inpatient units have attempted an integration of DBT skills training with individual psychodynamic therapy. Acute inpatient units may structure psychosocial treatment primarily around milieu and skills training, with individual therapy consisting of pharmacotherapy.

When skills training is offered outside of standard DBT, some modifications in the actual conduct of the skills training may be necessary. The exact modifications necessary depend somewhat on what kind of individual psychotherapy is being offered, as well as on the skills trainers' relationship with the individual psychotherapists.

When the Individual Psychotherapist Does Not Incorporate Skills Coaching Into Psychotherapy

Although some effort is made to integrate into current everyday life the new behaviors taught in skills training, the lack of time and the complexity of achieving such an integration require that each clients' individual therapist be actively engaged in helping the client apply the skills. The individual therapist is the day-to-day coach for the client.

One task of the DBT therapist is to apply the lens of behavioral skills when helping the client generate solutions to the problems she is confronting. Thus, when distress tolerance is the current treatment module (or a skill the therapist wishes the client to practice), problems may be viewed as ones where distress tolerance is needed. If interpersonal effectiveness is the focus, then the individual therapist may ask how the problem (or the solution) might be related to interpersonal actions. Generally, problems become "problems" because the events are associated with aversive emotional responses; one solution may be for the client to change her emotional response to the situation. An effective response may also be cast in terms of core mindfulness skills.

The ability to apply any one of the behavioral skills to any problematic situation is at once important and very difficult. Individual therapists must themselves know the behavioral skills inside and out and be able to think quickly in a session or a crisis. When the individual therapist is not familiar with the skills being taught, the solution is to do what is possible to inform the therapist. Strategies for this are discussed below.

The required active intervention and coaching may not be compatible with the individual psychotherapy a particular therapist is willing to engage in. Some therapists, for example, view helping clients learn new skillful behaviors as treating the "symptoms" instead of the "illness." In one setting starting DBT, individual psychotherapists (who were physicians) told clients that they had to get coaching from the nurses in how to replace maladaptive behaviors with skills. In my experience, clients with such therapists will need extra help in using the skills they are learning. They also need help in accepting the idea that the new skills are actually important, since their individual therapists are communicating that the "real therapy" is taking place with them.

Skills trainers can make a number of optional modifications to address these issues. They might set up an extra weekly training skills meeting where clients can get help in figuring out how to use their skills in troublesome life situations. But, people often need help at the moment they are in crisis. Skills training is like teaching basketball. Coaches not only conduct practice sessions during the week, they also attend the weekly game to help the players use what they were practicing all week. With outpatients, this is usually best done via telephone calls. In standard DBT, phone calls to skills training therapists are severely limited; almost all calls for help are directed to the clients' individual therapists. If an individual therapist does not take calls or give coaching, however, a skills trainer may decide to accept them at least when the reason for calling is to get such coaching.

On an inpatient unit, milieu staff members should learn the behavioral skills along with the clients. The staff members can then serve as coaches for the clients. One inpatient unit offers weekly skills consultation meetings. The meetings are run like academic office hours; clients can come any time during office hours for advice. (This variation was developed by Charles Swenson at Cornell Medical Center/New York Hospital at White Plains.) Ideally, clients can also call on one another for help. In another inpatient setting, one therapist teaches new skills; nursing staff members conduct regular homework review groups, where clients meet together to go over their attempts to practice new skills and get help with areas of difficulty; and individual ther-

apists reinforce use of skills by the clients (Barley et al., in press).

When the Individual Therapist Assumes That the Skills Trainer Will Help with Suicidal Crises

One of the key differences between DBT and many non-DBT individual therapies is the emphasis in DBT on modifying current maladaptive behaviors before ameliorating long-standing interpersonal conflicts and effects of early trauma and abuse. In fact, the DBT stance is that current high-risk suicidal behaviors (including all instances of parasuicide), therapy-interfering behaviors, and extreme quality-of-life-interfering behaviors must be modified before any sustained attempt is made to explore and resolve intensely disturbing interpersonal conflicts and previous abuse or trauma. Therapeutic exposure to stress requires, at a minimum, the ability to tolerate stress without resorting to suicide, parasuicide, extreme suicidal ideation, excessive therapy-interfering behaviors, or other extremely dysfunctional behaviors.

But—and this is the most important point—reduction of these maladaptive behaviors is *not* the goal specific to DBT skills training. Instead, skills training is focused on teaching *general* skills that the clients can apply to current problems in living. Application of these skills to current suicidal behavior, to behaviors interfering with therapy progress, and to other severely dysfunctional behaviors is not necessarily attempted in the first year by skills training therapists.

In fact, as I discuss later, discussion of current parasuicidal behavior is actively discouraged in skills training. The application of skills to very high-stress situations is not encouraged during early stages of skills training because it violates principles of shaping. Therapy-interfering behaviors, including extreme problems with skills training, are relegated to the individual therapists primarily because of time constraints in conducting skills training.

Problems with this skills training orientation arise when an individual therapist wants to ignore current maladaptive behaviors in favor of attending to long-term conflicts and early childhood experiences. Such an individual therapy emphasis, in the absence of a corresponding emphasis on coping skills, can lead to an exacerbation of current dysfunctional behaviors. The problems can be especially intense if the individual therapist misunderstands the goals of DBT skills training, mistaking it for a treatment focused directly on modifying current severely dysfunctional and suicidal behaviors.

In my experience, many non-DBT therapists do not

want to attend to the direct modification of current behaviors—an understandable reluctance if they are not behaviorally trained, and instead are relying on behaviorally oriented skills training therapy to do the job. Unfortunately, the skills training therapists in DBT are relying on the individual therapists in a similar manner. And therein lies the problem: In this case, no one is helping the clients modify their current style of coping with intensely disturbing experiences (posttraumatic stress, intrapsychic conflicts, interpersonal conflicts, or other major life stresses).

The problem is even worse when the individual therapists, relying on the skills training to develop the client's everyday coping abilities, begin to increase the stress level of individual therapy material while simultaneously reducing efforts at teaching coping skills. When this occurs, it seems reasonable to predict that the addition of DBT skills training to non-DBT individual therapy may be iatrogenic rather than therapeutic.

In these instances, it would seem necessary to conduct skills training for clients not receiving DBT individual therapy separately from skills training for the standard DBT clients. In this separate context, the pace should be slowed considerably, and a mechanism must be developed for discussion of suicidal behaviors in the skills training setting. One option is to schedule a second weekly session for just this purpose. Since such a discussion is often very disturbing to other clients, care must be taken to frame the discussion in a context of positive coping behaviors; to pay attention to silent clients who may be getting more suicidal without being able to express it; to plan work on individual coping strategies for after skills training meetings; and to make resources available after meetings for clients who become more suicidal during meetings.

All this is needed because, in my experience, suicidal individuals typically experience increased urges to engage in parasuicide when the topic of prior suicidal behavior (including urges) is discussed. It is precisely this escalation of risk, of course, that keeps many individual therapists from addressing the topic directly with their clients. Unfortunately, when the responsibility is shifted to the skills training therapists, the potential for trauma increases enormously.

Consultation Between Individual Psychotherapists and Skills Trainers

The problems discussed above sometimes result from poor communication between individual therapists and skills trainers. If the expectations of each group of therapists for the other are not spelled out and frequently reviewed, it is no wonder that the two treatments do not enhance each other. Among the most important aspects

of DBT are the supervision/consultation strategies (described in Chapter 13 of the text). These strategies require all DBT therapists to meet on a regular basis. The goals of these meetings are to share information and to keep therapists within the frame of DBT.

In my clinic, a supervision/consultation meeting is held each week for 2 hours. During the meeting, individual clients are discussed. The skills training therapists review for the individual therapists which skills are the current focus of group sessions. When necessary, the skills trainers actually teach the other therapists the skills. In this context, it is helpful for clients and decreases the potential for confusion if the individual and skills training therapists share a common language in discussing application of behavioral skills. Although consistency and conformity between various treating agents are not particularly valued in DBT, such consistency here can be useful, since the number of new skills to be learned is quite large. The weekly meetings increase this communality. In addition, any problems individual clients may be having in applying skills and/or interacting in skills training meetings are also mentioned. Individual therapists both consult with the skills trainers and take such information into account in planning the individual treatment.

My emphasis on the importance of meetings between individual and skills training therapists may seem to contradict the "consultation-to-the-patient" strategies, which are also integral to DBT. (See Chapter 13 of the text for a discussion of these strategies; they are also discussed briefly in Chapter 5 of this manual.) First, I must point out that these consultation strategies do require DBT therapists to walk a very fine line. The issues are somewhat complex.

When the therapeutic unit is defined as a group of people (including the individual and skills training therapists), a clinic, an inpatient unit, or some such entity where multiple therapists interact with particular clients in a coordinated treatment program, then consultation between therapists is essential, provided that the clients are informed of and consent to such collaboration. Applying the consultation strategies in these cases simply requires that therapists refrain from intervening with each other on *behalf* of a client. Thus, therapists must be careful not to fall into the trap of serving as intermediaries for a client.

A particularly difficult situation arises when a client's individual therapist works separately from the skills trainers and does not want to consult with them or does not have the time to do so. Can progress be made? The answer depends on the individual therapist's willingness and ability to assist the client in integrating skills independently. A therapist with good behavioral treatment skills could probably do a creditable job under some circumstances. First, the individual psychotherapist needs to elicit from the client sufficient information about the skills taught in skills training to be able to help the client apply the skills in troublesome areas. Second, the therapist needs to know and be able to apply the skills himself or herself; this is not as simple as it might seem. Third, the therapist needs to resist the temptation to rely on the skills trainer to conduct interventions aimed at reducing current suicidal and other severely dysfunctional behaviors. In my clinic, when skills training is offered to individuals with non-DBT individual therapists, we inform the therapists that we cannot accept their clients if they do not agree to coach the clients in applying skills. We then send the therapists our skills training materials. I discuss the issue of guidelines for handling suicidal and crisis behaviors at greater length later.

Group Leaders

In my experience, two leaders are essential for the conduct of group skills training in DBT. The primary reason for this is therapist burnout, which can happen very quickly to a therapist trying to conduct a group alone. The constant passivity, hopelessness, emotional vulnerability, and invalidation that pervade group skills training in the early months are all but impossible for a lone therapist to tolerate. The tendency of group members to withdraw emotionally in the face of group tension or conflict, including attempts by the therapist to "push" individual members along, creates a countertendency in the therapist to pull back, blame the victims, and then lash out at group members. Resisting this tendency alone is next to impossible over the long haul. The primary function of the second leader is to provide the dialectical balance and personal support that keeps the teetertotter (of acceptance and change; see Chapters 2 and 7 of the text) balanced for yet another week.

In our groups, we use a model of a primary group leader and a coleader. The functions of the two leaders during a typical session differ somewhat. The primary leader begins the meetings, conducts the initial behavioral analyses of homework practice, and presents new skills material. The primary group therapist is also responsible for the timing of the session, moving from person to person as time allows. Thus, the primary group leader has overall responsibility for skills acquisition.

The coleader's functions are more diverse. First, he or she mediates tensions that arise between members and the primary leader, providing a balance from which a synthesis can be created. Second, while the primary group leader is looking at the group as a whole, the coleader keeps a focus on each individual member, noting any need for individual attention and either addressing that need directly during group sessions or consulting with the primary leader during breaks. Third, the coleader serves as a coteacher and tutor, offering alternate explanations, examples, and so on.

Generally, if there is a "bad guy" it is the primary group leader, who enforces the group norms, and if there is a "good guy" it is the coleader, who always tries to see life from the point of view of the person who is "down." More often than not in a group meeting, though not always, the person who is "down" is a group member; thus, the "good guy" image emerges for the coleader. As long as both leaders keep the dialectical perspective of the whole, this division of labor and roles can be quite therapeutic. Obviously, it requires a degree of personal security on the part of both therapists if it is to work.

The DBT therapist supervision/consultation strategies can be especially important here. The supervision group serves as the third point providing the dialectical balance between the two coleaders, much as the coleader does between the primary leader and a group member in a group session. Thus, the function of the DBT supervision/consultation group is to highlight the truth in each side of an expressed tension, fostering reconciliation and synthesis.

3

Session Format and Starting Skills Training

Format and Organization of Sessions

There are a number of possible formats for skills training sessions. In my clinic, group skills training sessions last for 2½ hours, generally with a break in the middle. The format is reasonably consistent for the whole year. The first hour is devoted to opening rituals, followed by group members' sharing their attempts to practice behavioral skills (or lack thereof) during the preceding week, followed by a break. The second hour is devoted to presenting and discussing new skills. The last 15 minutes are for session "wind-down."

Some inpatient settings have split this format in two, holding two weekly sessions—one devoted to homework review and one devoted to new skills. This is a reasonable model on inpatient and day treatment units where staff members have some ability to persuade clients to attend both weekly sessions. In an outpatient setting, however, there is a danger that clients will not attend homework review sessions when they have not practiced any of their skills during the preceding week. Skills trainers will want to prevent that from occurring.

Other settings have tried to shorten the session time, usually from 2½ to 1½ hours. In our experience, 1½ hours simply does not give enough time for a group session. Even with 2½ hours, 50 to 60 minutes for homework review with eight group members gives each member from 6 to 8 minutes of group attention—not very much. Nor is 50 to 60 minutes for new material much time, either. Although group leaders can present a lot of material in that time, they also need time to do in-session practice of new skills, to discuss questions about the week's new content, to check skill comprehension with each member, and to go over new homework sheets

to be sure that clients understand how to do the practice and how to record it. Individual skills training can be accomplished in weekly 45- to 50-minute sessions.

The first 30–60 minutes of each *new* skills training module (remember that there are four) is spent in discussing the rationale for that particular module. (In an ongoing group, the time devoted to homework review is cut short the first session of each new module.) The leaders' task here is to convince the clients that the skills to be covered in the upcoming module are relevant to their lives; that if they improve these particular skills their lives will improve, and, most importantly, that they can actually learn the skills. The leaders often have to be creative in demonstrating how particular sets of skills apply to particular problems. The specific rationale for each module is described in Chapters 7–10.

Session Start-Up

At our group sessions we serve noncaffeinated coffee and tea (and usually snacks as well); the beginning of the group consists of each member's getting her coffee or tea and getting settled. The first task is to fill out whatever research or treatment evaluation scales we may be using at that point. If a member has missed one or more previous sessions, she is given a chance to tell the group where she has been. If missing sessions is a problem for such a person, some time (no more than 5 or so minutes) can be spent analyzing what interferes with her coming and how to overcome it. If there are group issues (e.g., announcements; not calling when missing, or coming late), they are dealt with at the beginning of the session. This brief attention to therapy-interfering behaviors is very important and should not be dropped.

Sharing of Practice Efforts/ Homework Review

The next phase of treatment is the sharing of efforts to practice the specific behavioral skills (mindfulness, interpersonal effectiveness, emotion regulation, distress tolerance) being taught. In our group sessions, the primary group leader goes around the circle and asks each member to share with the group what she has practiced during the preceding week. (In my experience, waiting for members to volunteer takes up too much time. However, I may let members decide who to start with in going around the circle.) Vocabulary can be very important here. Behaviorists are used to calling practice "homework," and therefore to asking clients about their "homework practice." Some of our clients like this terminology and prefer to think of skills training as a class they are taking, much like a college course. Others feel demeaned by the words, as if they are being treated like children in school, once again having to report to adults. A discussion of the semantics at the very beginning of treatment can be successful in defusing this issue.

The weekly sharing of homework practice efforts is an essential part of skills training. The sure knowledge that not only will each client be asked about her efforts to practice skills, but that not practicing will be analyzed in depth, serves as a powerful motivation for at least attempting to practice skills during the week. The norm of weekly *in vivo* practice is set and maintained during the sharing. Every client should be asked to share her experiences, even those who communicate extreme reluctance or aversion to the task. This part of the session is so important that its completion takes precedence over any other group task. To finish the sharing in the 50 to 60 minutes allotted takes very good time management skills on the part of the primary leader, as noted above. However, the usual absence of one or more clients together with the equally usual tendency of one or two each week to refuse to interact more than briefly, adds considerably to the time per person available for sharing.

Managing practice sharing requires enormous sensitivity on the part of the leaders. The tasks here are to prod each client gently to analyze her own behavior; to validate her difficulty and counter her tendency to judge herself negatively and hold tenaciously to impossibly high standards; and at the same time to help her develop, if needed, more effective skill strategies for the coming week. In addition, the leaders must be adept at alternating attention between analysis of the week's behaviors and focusing on the in-session attempts to describe, analyze, and solve problems. Fear of criticism or looking "stupid," shame, humiliation, embarrassment, self-hatred, and anger are common emotions interfering with the ability to engage in and profit from sharing. Deft handling of these emotions—combining validating strategies with problem-solving strategies, and irreverent communication with reciprocal communication— is the key to using practice sharing therapeutically.

If the client has practiced and the skills have worked, she should be supported and encouraged by the leaders. Other clients are asked to comment on the similarity of the practice or situation to their own lives. Client-to-client praise and encouragement are reinforced. It is very important to get each client to describe in detail her use of the skills in that particular week's problematic situations. The same amount of attention to detail must be given to the week's successes as to the week's difficulties. In addition, over time the leaders can use such information to identify the client's patterns in skill usage. This is especially important if a client is consistently reporting only one skill strategy. For example, in one of my groups I had a client who always tried to change problem situations as her primary method of emotion regulation. Although her skills at problem-solving situations were excellent and commendable, nonetheless, it was also important for her to learn other methods (e.g., cognitive restructuring, tolerating the situation, distracting herself, etc.). Not every problem situation can be changed. My experience is that when given a limited amount of time to share, borderline clients will almost always share their successes in using skills and will rarely want to describe their problems and failures. Thus, listening carefully to the successes is even more important than it might be with other populations.

When the Skills Did Not Help

If a client could not use the skills being taught, or reports using the skills but not getting any benefits from them, the leaders use problem-solving strategies to help the client analyze what happened, what went wrong, and how she could use the skills better next time. This is a very important opportunity for the leaders to model how to analyze situations and behaviors and how to apply self-management skills. Over time, it is important to encourage and reinforce clients in helping one another analyze and solve difficult problems.

When a Client Has Difficulty with Homework

During sharing, a client will often report that she did not practice at all during the preceding week. It would be an error to take the meaning of this comment at face value. On close examination, we often find that the client did practice; she just did not actually solve the problem. The discussion then turns to the issue of shaping and setting appropriate expectations. Often we find that the client does not have a complete understanding of how to practice the skill assigned. Or we may find that she does not understand many of the skills discussed previously but has been afraid to ask questions; in this instance, both the self-censoring of questions and the problem in homework practice should be discussed. Whenever possible, it is useful to encourage or ask other clients to help the person having difficulty. In the case of interpersonal effectiveness, we may ask another client to role-play how she would cope with the situation. Emotion regulation and distress tolerance do not lend themselves to demonstration, but other clients can share how they have coped (or would cope) with similar situations. Finally, a client who says she did not practice sometimes actually did practice, but did it either without realizing she had done it or by using skills learned outside skills training. This information can be missed completely if the patient's experiences during the week are not explored in enough depth.

Each skills training module contains a large number of specific behavioral skills. It is usually not such a good idea to present a lot of individual skills to be learned when conducting skills training; the idea is that it is better to learn a few skills well than a lot of skills poorly. However, in my experience with borderline individuals, presenting a lot of skills counteracts two problems. First, the need for a lot of skills suggests that the therapist is not oversimplifying the problems to be solved. Second, presenting a lot of skills works against a client's being able to say credibly that absolutely nothing works. If one thing doesn't work, the therapist can always suggest trying a different skill. With a lot of skills to draw from, the client's patience for resisting usually runs out before the therapist's patience for offering new skills to try. In addition, what works for whom is very individual. Leaders must be very careful, however, in assuming that the problem is that the client used the wrong skill. Inexperienced leaders often give up on a skill too easily. They may assume that the specific skill is not a good match for a specific group member when, in actuality, the client has not been applying the skill properly.

When a Client Did Not Do Any Homework Practice

When a client actually did not practice or attempt to do so, this absence is analyzed. Common reasons given by clients for not practicing are not wanting to, not remembering, and not having an occasion to. Rarely can they identify the situational factors influencing their lack of motivation, failure to remember, or inability to observe practice opportunities. Usually, the application of problem solving to the failure to practice reveals a pervasive difficulty in analyzing behavior (or the lack of behavior) and then applying learning principles to bring about desired changes. Borderline individuals tend to use

punishment, commonly in the form of self-denigration, as a form of behavior control. "If I didn't do it, I must not have wanted to do it" is a frequent comment. This comment, however, requires careful analysis: Motivational interpretations are often learned in previous therapies, even when they have little to do with reality.

Even if the problem *is* one of motivation, the question of what is interfering with motivation must be addressed. Failures in motivation and in memory offer important opportunities for the leaders to teach principles of behavioral management and learning. The goal over time is to use these principles to replace the judgmental theories based on willpower and mental illness that borderline individuals often hold. Failure to practice is a problem to be solved.

In a group setting, when a member has not attempted to practice during the preceding week, she will often not want to discuss why she didn't practice, and will ask the primary leader simply to go on to the next person. In my experience, it is essential that the leader not be convinced to do this. The analysis of not doing homework can be very important. In the case of the person who is avoiding the topic because of fear or shame, it offers a chance to practice "opposite action," a skill taught in the emotion regulation module. It also offers other group members an opportunity to practice their own behavior management and problem-solving skills within the context of the group. It is, of course, important that the leader resist the temptation to collude with a client in punishing herself for not practicing.

Break

Most clients get restless after about an hour or so of a group session. We usually take a 10- or 15-minute break at about the halfway mark. Members can get a refill of coffee or tea, and a snack if provided. Most clients go to the smoking area or go outside for fresh air. This part of the session is important because it provides an unstructured period of time for group clients to interact. Generally, the group leaders stay near but somewhat apart from group clients. Group cohesion, independent of the leaders, is thus fostered. If a member needs individual attention, it is given at this point. One of our main problems has been that clients having a hard time at a session often leave during the break. We have found it advisable to be particularly alert to anyone who may be leaving, so that intervention can be attempted before she walks out.

Presentation of New Material

The hour after the break is devoted to the presentation and discussion of new skills (or, if necessary the review of ones already covered). The content and manner of skills presentation for each module are discussed in Chapters 7–10.

Wind-Down

A time at the end of a skills training session for winding down seems particularly important for borderline clients. These sessions are almost always emotionally charged and painful for some. Borderline individuals are acutely aware of the negative effects of their own skill deficits. Without emotion regulation skills of their own, clients can be in great emotional difficulty following a session, especially if nothing is done to help them regulate their affect and end or "close up" the session, so to speak.

A wind-down period also provides a time for clients who have dissociated during the session, usually because of painful memories, to come back into the session before parting. I was alerted to this need during my first DBT skills training group. After several months it came up in a group discussion that almost every member of the group was going out drinking after the meetings as a means of affect control. Skills trainers will often find that topics that seem very innocuous are actually very stress-provoking for borderline individuals. For example, a group member once became extremely emotional and disorganized as I was introducing the interpersonal effectiveness module and the fact that one task of the module would be to learn to say no effectively. She was currently enmeshed in a group of drug dealers who frequently raped her. She didn't say no because the group was her meal ticket.

I have used several methods of winding down. The most popular with our group members is the process-observing wind-down. In this method, we spend about 15 minutes sharing our observations of how things went in the session. Members may offer observations about themselves, one another, the leaders, or the group as a whole. Although the leaders may have to model such observations at the beginning of the year, members usually pick up on the method rapidly. As time progresses, we find that members usually become quite astute observers and describers of one another's behavior, progress, mood changes, and apparent difficulties. At times, the leaders may facilitate more in-depth observations and comments by asking general questions about observations (e.g., "What do you make of that?"). Or the leaders may encourage a member to check out an observation, especially when an observation involves an inference about another's feelings, mood state, or opinion. Another important leaders' task is to draw out members who do not spontaneously offer an observation. During wind-down, each member should be encouraged

to offer at least one observation, even if that observation is simply that it is difficult to offer an observation.

Although the process-observing wind-down may be the most popular, it is also the wind-down with the most potential for creating problems. These problems almost always have to do with the observation period's getting out of control of the leader and ending in overly critical observations, in escalating responses to critical feedback, and occasionally in members' storming out and refusing ever to come back. This can be a special problem if more experienced or advanced clients (e.g., those who have gone through several skills training modules) are mixed with clients beginning in skills training. The more advanced clients may be ready for much more process than new clients can tolerate. The process-observing wind-down is a natural place for them to begin to try out more confrontational comments. I discuss the problems of too much process work in first-year skills training groups more thoroughly in Chapter 5 of this manual.

A second wind-down method consists of leading clients through relaxation, visualization, meditation, and breathing exercises. The focus here is on observing internal events (body sensation, breath, thoughts, feelings, etc.). The exercise is begun by asking clients to get in a comfortable position in their chairs, with their backs straight. My experience is that borderline individuals are often so self-conscious about their bodies that for the first several months of doing these exercises. many will not move into a position of sitting up in their chairs. With time and patience, however, most clients eventually begin to enter fully into the exercises. They are then instructed either to close their eyes or to keep them only partially opened. Once again, several clients can be expected to have difficulty closing their eyes in the session; nor is it necessary that they do so. For those keeping their eyes open, we ask them to find a place to look that is not too distracting. Third, clients are instructed to focus their attention on their breathing, as they take three very deep breaths, hold each for a second or two, and then let each out in a long, slow, exhalation. The focus on the three breaths is a vehicle for settling down and directing attention to inner experiences.

At this point, a skills trainer directs the clients in a specific observing exercise. The possibilities are too innumerable to describe here. We may do an abbreviated relaxation exercise that consists of tensing and relaxing various body muscle groups. The modification we make is that the trainer consistently focuses the clients' attention on observing their internal body reactions and sensations. Or we may do a sensate focus exercise in which the trainer instructs clients to focus their attention on various body parts, noticing the sensations that arise in each. An exercise that I have found useful is one that combines sensate focusing ("Can you feel your arm resting on the arm rest?") and visualization ("Can you see a rose, just opening, in your mind's eye?"). Imaginal exercises may include imagining lying on a warm beach, drifting on a cloud, being a pebble lazily floating to the bottom of the ocean or some other similarly relaxing scene. Meditation exercises may focus on repeating a simple word over and over (such as the word "one") or on counting thoughts that go through the mind or breaths. In meditation it is particularly important to instruct clients to go back gently to the exercise, letting go of judging, whenever they find their minds drifting.

In my experience, internal observation exercises such as those described above must be very brief at the beginning, not more than 5 minutes. Also, care must be taken to counter unrealistic performance expectations. For example, the drifting of attention in meditation is to be expected and accepted, not resisted. The idea is, simply, to keep coming back. Attempts to visualize may not be successful; people differ in their capacity for visual imagery. The key idea is to observe and accept whatever happens.

As the discussion of core mindfulness skills in Chapter 7 indicates, these wind-down exercises involve practicing the skills of observing and taking a nonjudgmental stance. Process observing also includes practice in describing. Relaxation and meditation provide practice in focusing on one thing in the moment.

Beginning Skills Training

Building Relationships

Use of the therapeutic relationship strategies (see Chapter 15 of the text) is particularly important at the start of skills training. In a group context, among the first tasks of the group leaders are to enhance the bonding between group clients and the leaders, and to begin the process of building group cohesion. We have found it useful to have the leaders call each new group member a few days before the first skills training meeting to remind her of the session, clarify directions, and communicate looking forward to meeting her. It is also a good time for the leaders to address last-minute fears and plans to drop out before even starting (not uncommon plans for borderline clients).

The leaders should arrive a few minutes early before each group meeting, including the first, to greet clients and interact briefly but individually with each one. For reluctant and/or fearful clients, this can be a soothing experience. It also offers an opportunity for leaders to hear concerns and refute plans to leave early. We try to confine these individual interactions to the context of group mingling, in order to keep the essential identity of group rather than individual therapy. This issue is discussed further below.

As might be expected, group members are very timid and fearful during the first meeting. Appropriate behavior is not clear, and the trustworthiness of group clients is doubtful. We generally begin by going around the group and asking each person to give her name, how she heard about the group, and any information about herself she cares to share. The group leaders also give information about themselves and how they came to be leading the group.

The next task of skills trainers is to help clients see the relevance of a skills training model to their own lives. An overview of the skills training treatment year is given; a theory of BPD and suicidal behaviors that stresses the role of inadequate skills is presented; and the format for the upcoming sessions is described. Discussion is elicited at each point about the relevance of the material to the client's own experiences. A handout illustrating the relationship between characteristics of BPD and skills training is distributed and discussed (see Chapter 6 of this manual for details); usually I also write this on the blackboard in the therapy room.

It is essential here for the skills trainer to communicate an expectancy that the treatment will be effective at helping the clients improve the quality of their own lives. The treatment must be "marketed" to clients. (See Chapters 9 and 14 of the text for further discussion of marketing therapy to clients and eliciting commitments.) At this time I usually make the point that DBT is not a suicide prevention program, but a life enhancement program. It is not our idea to get people to live lives not worth living, but rather to help them build lives they actually want to live. Validation and didactic strategies (see Chapters 8 and 9 of the text) are the primary treatment vehicles here.

Skills Training Rules

It is important to make the rules of skills training explicit at the very beginning, as well as to discuss possible misconceptions about how to "get around" the rules. Presentation of the rules offers an opportunity for the skills trainers to specify and obtain agreement to the treatment contract from each client. In a group context, it can be useful after discussion of the rules to go around the room and ask each group member for an individual commitment to abide by them. My experience is that the presentation and discussion of rules can usually be accomplished during the first session. In an open group, the rules should be discussed each time a new member enters the group. Often it is a good idea to have old members explain the rules to new members.

The skills trainers need to be aware that the discussion of rules is an important part of the treatment process, not a precursor to the process. As such, it will be repeated over and over as skills training progresses. Presentation of rules in an authoritarian way will probably alienate some clients, especially those for whom issues of control are important. Rules I have found useful are discussed below. (They are also presented to clients in a handout; see Chapter 6.)

1. Clients Who Drop Out of Therapy Are Out of Therapy

Clients who miss 4 weeks of scheduled skills training sessions in a row have dropped out of therapy and cannot re-enter for the duration of the time in their treatment contract. For example, if a client has contracted for 1 year, but misses 4 weeks in a row during the sixth month, then she is out for the next 6 months or so. At the end of the contracted time, she can negotiate with the skills trainer(s) (and the group, if she was in one and it is continuing) about readmission. There are no exceptions to this rule.

The rule for skills training, thus, is the same as the rule for individual DBT psychotherapy. We mention that although it is technically possible to repeatedly miss three sessions in a row and come to the fourth, that would be a violation of the spirit of the rule. In our advanced groups, the rules for what constitute dropping out vary, and are adopted by group consensus. For example, in one group, three "unexcused" absences in any 4-month period are the equivalent of dropping out of the group. In all groups, we make it crystal clear at the beginning— either by presenting the rules as in first-year groups, or by mutual decision making in ongoing groups—how one goes about dropping out of therapy.

The message communicated is that we expect everyone to come to skills training sessions each week. Presentation of this rule offers an opportunity to discuss what constitutes an acceptable reason for missing a session. Not being in the mood, nonserious illness, social engagements, fear, beliefs that "No one in the group likes me," and so forth, do not qualify; serious illness, very important events, and unavoidable trips out of town do.

In our first research project with 24 clients in standard DBT group skills training plus DBT individual therapy, we had a 1-year dropout rate of 16.4%—considerably below the 50–80% dropout rate we expected. In a second study, we had 12 clients receiving DBT skills training plus ongoing non-DBT individual psychotherapy in the community. There was a 27% dropout rate at 1 year, which again was lower than the expected 50% rate. I suspect that our emphasis on a time-limited commitment and the clarity of the rules about how to drop out are crucial in our low dropout rate. The rule clarity

is important for two reasons. First, it tells clients that if they miss 1, 2, or 3 weeks in a row, even without calling, they are still welcome back. They know ahead of time that their behavior is not totally unexpected and they will not be terminated from skills training. Second, it makes it more difficult for people just to slide out of therapy without quite realizing they are doing it. Each week, clients are aware of where the line is between staying in skills training and dropping out.

2. Each Client Has to Be in Ongoing Individual Therapy

The fact that skills training in DBT is designed to be an adjunct to individual psychotherapy for borderline clients is presented clearly at the beginning of therapy. Clients may switch individual therapists during the course of skills training, but they cannot go 4 consecutive weeks without a session with an individual therapist. Four consecutive weeks of no individual therapy is considered dropping out of skills training. When clients are in our standard DBT program (group skills training plus individual therapy), dropping out of individual therapy (unless we have another individual therapist available or can find one in the community) is tantamount to dropping out of group skills training, and therefore out of the total treatment program.

Individual therapy is needed for several reasons. First, with a group of eight seriously suicidal clients, it would be extraordinarily difficult for the skills trainers to handle the crisis calls that might be needed. The caseload is simply too large. Second, in a skills oriented program meeting only once a week, there is not much time to attend to individual process issues that may come up. Nor is there time to adequately help each individual integrate the skills into her life. Some need much more time than do others on particular skills, and the need to adjust the pace to the average needs makes it very likely that without outside attention everyone will fail to learn at least some of the skills.

This early beginning emphasis on highlighting the likely need of each participant for extra help in mastering the skills is very important later when the clients run into difficulty. It is all too easy for the trainers to overestimate the ease of learning skills; such overestimation sets the clients up for later disillusionment and hopelessness.

This is also a good time to communicate that, in general, the discussions will focus on the skills being learned and on how each client can use the skills in her own life. Thus, with brief exceptions, discussion of current life problems and crises will not be encouraged. It is crucial, however, that the skills trainers validate the need to discuss problems with someone. They are important and serious; thus, this is another reason for individual therapy.

In a group context, it is essential at this point that the leaders discuss the difference between a skills training group and other group therapies. Many individuals look forward to a group where they can share with individuals like themselves. Although there is much sharing in the group, it is not unlimited and it is focused on practicing skills, not on whatever crises may have occurred during the week. Many participants have never been in any kind of behavior therapy, much less a skills-oriented group. My experience is that the difference cannot be stressed too much. Often the clients have had an enormous amount of nonbehavioral therapy in which they have been taught various "necessary ingredients" for therapeutic change—ingredients often not focused on extensively in skills training. In every group we have conducted so far, one or more clients have gotten angry about their inability to talk about "what is really important" in the group. For one client, talking about whatever comes to mind was so firmly associated with the process of therapy that she refused to acknowledge that skills training could be a form of therapy. Needless to say, there was much friction with her in the group.

The requirement for individual therapy can be quite formidable at times. In our experience, it is not uncommon for individual therapists in the community to get pushed past their limits and then to terminate therapy precipitously with borderline clients. When this happens, it can be extraordinarily difficult to find an individual therapist willing to work with such clients, especially with those who are mourning the loss of previous therapists. This is especially problematic when the clients cannot afford to pay the high fees often charged by professionals who are experienced enough to be helpful. Unfortunately, many public health clinics are so understaffed that they cannot provide individual psychotherapy, or clients may have already burned out their local clinics. In these cases, the skills training leaders often must function as short-term backup crisis therapists and assist the clients in finding appropriate individual therapists.

3. Clients Are Not to Come to Sessions under the Influence of Drugs or Alcohol

As with the confidentiality rule, the value of the third rule is reasonably self-evident; thus there is little need for extensive discussion of it. However, it does offer an opportunity to discuss the emotional pain that skills training attendance is likely to cause much of the time. Accurate expectations are essential here to head off demoralization. Once again, the skills trainers can suggest that as clients learn emotion regulation skills, they will be better able to cope with the stress of skills training. Because it is so important in treating this population, this topic is discussed in more detail at a later point.

4. Clients Are Not to Discuss Past (Even if Immediate) Parasuicidal Behaviors with Other Clients Outside of Sessions

The reasons for the fourth rule are several. First, at every point in DBT a major objective is to diminish the opportunity for reinforcement of suicidal behaviors. The usual (though not invariable) reactions from other clients to hearing of parasuicidal behaviors are sympathy, interest, and concern. Thus, just as in individual therapy, clients may not call their therapists *after* a parasuicidal act, in skills training they must agree not to call or communicate with one another after the fact. In addition, my experience is that communications about parasuicide elicit a strong imitation effect among borderline individuals. Hearing about another's cutting, overdosing, or the like often elicits an urge to imitate it, which can be difficult to resist. Our group members usually very much welcome this rule. Before I instituted this rule, clients often complained that once they had given up the behavior themselves, it was very scary to listen to others describing their parasuicidal episodes. Discussion during sessions is acceptable, although not encouraged, because it offers an opportunity for clients to examine alternate methods of solving the problem leading up to the suicidal behavior.

5. Clients Who Call One Another for Help When Feeling Suicidal Must Be Willing to Accept Help from the Person Called

It is not acceptable for a client to call someone, say "I am going to kill myself," and then refuse to let the person she called help. As noted in Chapter 8 of this manual, the inability to ask for help appropriately is a special problem for borderline individuals. Thus, this rule begins the process in the skills training context of teaching how to reach out to peers for help when needed. Like the fourth rule, this rule is usually a relief to clients. The rule itself was suggested by one of our group clients. Before the rule, we occasionally had instances of a member's calling another member in desperate emotional pain, obliquely threatening suicide, extracting a promise of confidentiality out of the one called, and then hanging up after no apparent progress in the call. The helper was left with a very difficult dilemma. If she really cared about the caller, she would do something to save her life. Yet she clearly couldn't do anything herself, and if she asked for outside help she was violating a confidence. The resulting helplessness and anguish were enormous.

However, when this problem was discussed, group members made it very clear to me that if I put in a rule that they could not promise to keep such a confidence, they would simply stop asking for help from one another. One of the strengths of group skills training, however, is that members often build a strong supportive community among themselves. At times, they are the only ones able to really understand their mutual experiences. Since everyone's suicidal and self-injurious desires are public, members need not be ashamed to ask one another for help. Not only is the opportunity for problem solving helpful to the caller, but the helper has a chance to practice generating problem solutions and reasons for living. In addition, and a point that therapists should note, such calls offer group members a structured chance to practice observing their own limits on how much help they are willing to give.

6. Information Obtained during Sessions, as Well as the Names of Clients, Must Remain Confidential

The importance of the confidentiality rule is self-evident. What may not be obvious is that the rule extends to "gossiping" outside of sessions. The general notion here is that interpersonal problems between or among clients should be dealt with by the persons involved, either inside or outside of sessions. There are two exceptions to the confidentiality rule. First, clients can discuss what happens in skills training sessions with their individual therapists; this exception is important so that they can maximize the benefits of the therapy. But, clients are cautioned not to reveal other clients' last names unless absolutely necessary. The other exception has to do with the risk of suicide. If one client believes that another is likely to commit suicide, she can and should summon help.

7. Clients Who Are Going to Be Late or Miss a Session Should Call Ahead of Time

The seventh rule serves several purposes. First, it is a courtesy to let skills trainers know not to wait for latecomers before starting. Although we have a general rule in our groups of starting on time, it is difficult not to hold off on important material or announcements for the first few minutes, in the expectation that missing clients will show up any minute. This is a special problem in those weeks where only one or two clients are present at the beginning. Second, it introduces an added response cost for being late and communicates to clients that promptness is desirable. Finally, it gives information as to why a client is not present.

In a group context, when a person does not come to a session and gives no explanation ahead of time, group members (including the leaders) almost always start worrying about the welfare of the absent member. Suicide is one of the first explanations that jumps to mind (although we have not had an unexplained absence to date because of suicide); emotional distress is another possibility; hospitalization is a third. Sometimes, however, clients miss for reasons having nothing to do with problems. Thus, not calling causes unnecessary worry for the group members. Just the fact that others will worry is often news to some group members; for others, the worry is a source of emotional support and may reinforce not calling. In any case, the rule offers a vehicle for addressing the behavior. Presentation of the rule is an opportunity to discuss the need for courtesy and empathy to feelings of other group members, as well as the responsibility of each member to contribute to group cohesion.

8. Clients May Not Form Private Relationships Outside of Training Sessions

The key word in the eighth rule is "private." The meaning of this rule is that clients may not form relationships outside of the sessions that they then cannot discuss in the sessions. DBT encourages outside-of-session relationships among group clients. In fact, the support that members can give one another with daily problems in living is one of the strengths of group DBT. The model here is similar to that of Alcoholics Anonymous and other self-help groups, where calling one another between meetings, socializing, and offering mutual support are viewed as therapeutic. Encouragement of such relationships, however, provides the possibility for interpersonal conflict that is inherent in any relationship. For a group of individuals selected partially because they often have interpersonal difficulties, this possibly may be either an opportunity or a liability. The key is whether interpersonal problems that arise outside of the sessions can be discussed in the sessions (or, if that is too difficult, with the leaders). To the extent that such issues can be discussed and appropriate skills can be applied, a relationship can be advantageous. Troubles arise when a relationship cannot be discussed and problems increase to such an extent that one member finds it difficult or impossible to attend meetings, either physically or emotionally.

Presentation of this rule alerts each member that leaders will respect the rights and needs of each member equally. It provides somewhat of a protective balance, communicating that it is unacceptable for one member to demand complete confidentiality about problems from another member. This is especially crucial when it comes to plans for destructive behavior, important information that one person lies about in meetings, and other situations creating an untenable awkwardness for one member of the pair.

9. Sexual Partners May Not Be in Skills Training Together

Assignment of current sexual partners to different groups at the onset is, of course, the responsibility of the group leaders. Thus, this rule functions to alert group members that if they enter into a sexual relationship, one member of the pair will have to drop out. To date we have had two sexual relationships begin among group members; both created enormous difficulties for the partners involved. In one case, the initiating partner broke off the relationship against the wishes of the other, making it very hard for the rejected partner to come to group sessions. In the other, one member was seduced reluctantly, leading to trauma and tension in the group. Generally, this rule is clear to everyone involved. Without the rule, however, dealing with an emerging sexual relationship between clients is very tricky, since post hoc application of rules is unworkable with borderline individuals.

4

Application of Structural Strategies and Skills Training Procedures to Psychosocial Skills Training

DBT therapy strategies are grouped into five major categories: (1) dialectical strategies, (2) core strategies, (3) stylistic strategies, (4) case management strategies, and (5) integrative strategies. "Strategies" are coordinated activities, tactics, and procedures that a therapist employs to achieve treatment goals—in this case, the acquisition of psychosocial skills. "Strategies" also describe the role and focus of the therapist and may refer to coordinated responses that the therapist should give to a particular problem presented by a client.

The core strategies of problem solving and validation, together with dialectical strategies, form the essential components of DBT. Stylistic strategies specify interpersonal and communication styles compatible with the therapy. Case management strategies specify how the therapist interacts with and responds to the social network in which the client is enmeshed. Integrative strategies outline how to handle specific problem situations that ordinarily come up in treating borderline individuals, such as problems in the therapeutic relationship, suicidal behaviors, therapy-interfering behaviors, and ancillary treatments. Structural strategies, a special category of integrative strategies, have to do with structuring therapy time. Some strategies will be used much more often than others, and it is possible that one or more of the strategies will be needed only rarely. Some strategies may not be necessary or appropriate for a given skills training session, and the pertinent combination of strategies may change over time.

The structuring of treatment time (including the treatment targets or goals addressed) is the major factor differentiating DBT psychosocial skills training from

DBT individual psychotherapy. In skills training, the therapy agenda is set by the behavioral skill to be taught; the agenda is set before a client shows up for the session. In individual DBT psychotherapy, the agenda is set by a client's behavior since the last session and within the current session; the agenda is open until the client shows up for the session. Although in my clinic we conduct skills training in groups, as I have said before, it can be done individually. (I am also quite sure that DBT psychotherapy could be conducted in a group context, although I have not written a guide for that yet.) In this chapter, I first discuss how to use DBT structural strategies in skills training. (The other major strategies are reviewed briefly in the next chapter.)

Next, I review the skills training procedures discussed in Chapter 11 of the main text. In the context of DBT as a whole, skills training procedures constitute one of four sets of change procedures; the other three are contingency, exposure-based, and cognitive modification procedures. Skills training procedures, as their name suggests, will be the "meat" of interventions in psychosocial skills training. However—and this is important—it is impossible to do a competent job in skills training without an understanding of how to make contingencies work in psychotherapy (contingency procedures), how to manage exposure to threatening material and situations (exposure-based procedures), and how to deal with maladaptive expectancies, assumptions, and beliefs (cognitive modification procedures). In most senses, these procedures cannot be pulled apart from the implementation of skills training procedures; I do so here and in the text only for the sake of exposition. (I briefly review the application of these procedures to psychosocial skills training in the next chapter.)

Structural Strategies

Structural strategies have to do with how DBT as a whole is started and ended, as well as how individual skills training sessions are begun and ended. They also have to do with how time is structured during treatment and during individual sessions. There are five sets of structural strategies: (1) contracting strategies, (2) session-beginning strategies, (3) targeting strategies, (4) session ending strategies, and (5) terminating strategies. These are discussed in detail in Chapter 14 of the text.

Contracting Strategies

There are six specific contracting strategies: (1) conducting pretreatment assessment; (2) presenting the biosocial theory of borderline behavior patterns and the role of skills in these behaviors; (3) orienting the client(s) to specifics of skills training; (4) developing a collaborative commitment to do psychosocial skills training together, (5) assessing specific skill deficits, and (6) beginning to develop a therapeutic relationship. All of these steps should be gone through on two occasions: During initial individual interviews with each client before she is admitted to skills training, and during the first session of each skills training module. In addition, as in individual DBT, therapists can expect to repeat many of the strategies over and over as treatment progresses.

Pretreatment Individual Session

All potential members of a skills training program, whether it is conducted individually or in a group, should have one or more meetings with the skills training therapist (and the coleader, in the case of a group) to decide together whether skills training is appropriate and, if so, what form the training should take. Such a session should begin with reasonably thorough assessment (the first strategy listed above), including diagnostic interviewing as needed, at least to assess BPD. The session should also include some assessment of the individual's psychosocial skills, as necessary (the fifth strategy above); this can be done either informally or formally using structured behavioral assessments. Following assessment, the therapist should briefly present the biosocial theory of BPD (the second strategy above), which is discussed briefly in Chapter 1 of this manual and in detail in Chapter 2 of the text. In the standard DBT program, these three steps will have been covered as part of acceptance into the total treatment and do not

need to be repeated in full in this individual meeting.

It is very important, however, to go through the other three strategies, even if they have already been covered by intake personnel or other members of the treatment team. The individual pretreatment interview should orient the client to specifics of skills training (the third strategy listed above)—how the group (if there is a group) will function, and the client's role as well as the therapist's in treatment. I discuss orienting to skills training in more detail later in this chapter. The therapist should also decide whether skills training, either individually or in group therapy, appears appropriate for this client, and if so should make a commitment to accepting this client (the fourth strategy above). Most important, the therapist should follow all of the DBT guidelines on obtaining an initial therapy commitment; these are outlined and discussed in Chapters 9 and 14 of the text. This point cannot be over-stressed. It is impossible to get too much commitment! The skills trainer should not assume that other therapists (e.g., the individual psychotherapist or the intake interviewer in a clinic setting) have gotten the commitment needed. The pretreatment session is also a good opportunity to begin developing a personal therapeutic relationship with the client (the sixth strategy; see Chapters 14 and 15 of the text for more on this topic).

First Skills Training Session

The first session of skills training has been discussed in Chapter 3 of this manual; it is also outlined (including what to say, etc.) in Chapter 6. As those chapters indicate, the third, fourth and sixth contracting strategies discussed above are repeated in the first skills training session. Furthermore, in group psychosocial skills training, the group leaders should get commitments from the group as a whole as well as public commitments from each individual member. The rationale here is that public commitments are more powerful than private commitments. All of the commitment strategies outlined in Chapter 9 of the text should be employed.

Session-Beginning and Session-Ending Strategies

How to begin and end skills training sessions has been discussed in Chapter 3 of this manual and is also outlined in Chapter 6. The principles here are the same as in individual DBT, although the attention to ending sessions appropriately is much more structured in group skills training than in individual psychotherapy. A therapist who is conducting skills training individually should follow the session-beginning and session-ending guidelines in Chapter 14 of the text, except that if there is a need to repair relationship difficulties at the beginning of a session, only a limited amount of time should be spent at it. If possible, the therapist should help the client use her distress tolerance crisis survival strategies (see Chapter 10 of this manual) to distract from the need for further repair, do skills training, and get back to repair at the next individual psychotherapy meeting.

Terminating Strategies

It is very important to remember that terminating a 1-year psychosocial skills training program even in a group context, can be just as difficult for clients and therapists alike as terminating an intense, individual psychotherapy relationship. This can be very easy to forget. On the surface, at least, it may not appear that the attachment is as strong in group skills training. In my experience, at least, people who are more familiar with individual therapy than with group therapy tend to underestimate the degree of attachment group members have to one another, to the group as a whole, and to the group leaders. Therapists must be careful to pay as much attention to terminating in skills training as they do in other types of therapy, such as individual psychotherapy. All the termination strategies outlined in Chapter 14 of the text should be used. Steps for terminating skills training modules are outlined in Chapter 6 of this manual.

Targeting Strategies

The DBT targeting strategies have to do with how time is structured during skills training sessions and what topics receive attention. They were developed to reflect the DBT emphasis on hierarchical organization of treatment targets and to insure that therapists attend to the hierarchical ordering necessary in DBT. Implementing the targeting strategies requires an integration of almost all the DBT treatment strategies. It can be extremely difficult in the first stage of DBT (see Chapter 6 of the text for a discussion of stages), because often both clients and therapists do not want to attend to skills training. Work on the therapeutic process, having "heart-to-heart" talks, resolving real-life crisis, and so forth can all be more reinforcing (for both therapists and clients) than the sometimes mundane task of working on general psychosocial skills.

The rationale for the targeting strategies, and various objections to and difficulties with them, are discussed quite extensively in Chapters 5 and 6 of the text. It bears repeating here, however, that a therapist who ignores the targeting strategies is not doing DBT skills training. That is, in DBT *what* is discussed is as important as *how* it is discussed. Difficulties getting the client to go along with the targeting strategies should be treated

as problems to be solved (see discussion of the therapy-interfering behavior protocol in Chapter 15 of the text). A therapist who is having trouble following the targeting strategies, (a not unlikely problem) should bring up the topic in the next supervision/consultation team meeting. (Chapter 13 of the text discusses the role of such meetings in DBT.)

Because I have already discussed the rationale for targeting at such length in the text, I do not go through it again here. Skills training targets are, in order of importance: (1) stopping behaviors very likely to destroy therapy, (2) skill acquisition, and strengthening and generalization, and (3) reducing therapy-interfering behaviors. Target priorities indicate what is most important to address during sessions; in effect, they set the agenda. The agenda for skill acquisition, strengthening, the generalization is outlined in Chapters 6–10 of this manual. Although this agenda is the impetus for skills training in the first place, it must be set aside when behaviors emerge that are likely to destroy the treatment, either for a specific person or (in a group context) for the group as a whole. In contrast to DBT individual psychotherapy, however, behaviors that slow down progress in therapy (rather than threaten to destroy it altogether) are last rather than second in the hierarchy.

A comparison of this hierarchy with the hierarchy for DBT as a whole and for individual psychotherapy (described in Chapters 5 and 6 of the text) indicates the role of skills training in the total scheme of things. A therapist who is conducting both the individual psychotherapy and skills training for a particular client must be very clear about which targets take priority in which treatment modes. Maintaining the distinction between modes is one of the keys to successful DBT.

Stopping Behaviors Likely to Destroy Therapy

The highest-priority target is stopping client behaviors that, when and if they occur, pose a serious threat to the continuation of therapy. The behavior has to be *very serious* to be considered this high in priority. The emphasis here is a simple matter of logic: If therapy is destroyed, other targets cannot be achieved. The object here is to maintain the skills training sessions. Included in this target are violent behaviors, such as throwing objects, pounding loudly or destructively on things, and hitting or verbally attacking other clients during group therapy sessions. (Verbal attacks on the therapists are not considered therapy-destroying behavior.) Parasuicidal acts (e.g., cutting or scratching wrists, picking off scabs so that bleeding starts, taking excessive medications) and suicide crisis behaviors (e.g., threatening suicide in a credible manner and then storming out of the session) during group sessions (including breaks) are also not allowed. Also included are behaviors that make it impossible for anyone to concentrate, focus, or hear what is going on (e.g., yelling, hysterical crying, loud moaning, or constant out-of-turn talking). At times, an interpersonal problem among group members or between members and leaders, or a structural problem in the way skills training is delivered, may be so serious that if it is not attended to skills training will fall apart. Or one member may not be able to come back to skills training because of an interpersonal clash, hurt feelings, excessive hopelessness, or the like. In these cases, repairing the problem should be targeted. A therapist may attend to an individual problem by phone between sessions or before or after sessions, if not in the session itself. When we had a suicide in one of our groups, we dropped the skills acquisition agenda for the next several weeks to process group members' feelings about the suicide. Finally, a united rebellion of the clients against the therapists is also considered a top-priority target (as is a rebellion of the therapists against the clients).

The skills trainer's goal is to stop therapy-destructive behaviors and resolve rips in the therapeutic fabric as quickly and as efficiently as possible. Any further work on the destructive behaviors is left for the individual or primary psychotherapist to handle. (Behaviors that interfere with any mode of DBT treatment are considered therapy-interfering behaviors from the point of view of the DBT individual therapist.) Although teaching clients interpersonal effectiveness, emotion regulation, distress tolerance, or mindfulness skills may be useful in reducing the destructive behavior, a number of other treatment strategies (e.g., utilization of aversive contingencies) may be necessary to bring these behaviors under control quickly.

When suicide crisis behaviors occur (which by definition suggest a high likelihood of impending suicide), skills training therapists do the absolute minimum crisis intervention necessary and then as quickly as possible turn the problem over to the individual therapist. Except to determine whether medical care is needed immediately, reports of previous parasuicidal acts are given almost no attention by skills trainers. "Remember to tell your therapist," is the modal response. The one exception, as noted above, is when these behaviors in a group context become destructive to continuation of therapy for other group members. They are then targeted directly in the skills training group sessions. The general principle is that all therapists other than the individual psychotherapist treat a client in a suicidal crisis like a student who gets deathly ill in school. The nearest relative (in this case, the individual therapist) is called. A skills trainer who is also the individual client's therapist should turn the problem over to himself or herself, so to speak, *after* the skills training session. Unless it is impossible to

do otherwise, skills training should not be interrupted to attend to suicidal crisis.

Attention to suicidal ideation and communications during skills training is limited to helping the client figure out how to apply the DBT skills currently being taught to the suicidal feelings and thoughts. During mindfulness training, the focus may be on observing and describing the urge to engage in parasuicide or thoughts of suicide as these come and go. During distress tolerance training, the emphasis may be on tolerating the pain or using crisis intervention skills to cope with the situation. During emotion regulation training, the focus may be on observing, describing, and trying to change the emotions related to suicidal urges. In an interpersonal effectiveness framework, the emphasis may be on saying no or asking for help skillfully. The same strategy is used when the client discusses life crises, problems interfering with the quality of her life, or previous traumatic events in her life. Everything is grist for the skill application mill, so to speak.

Skill Acquisition, Strengthening, and Generalization

With very few exceptions, most of skills training time is devoted to acquisition, strengthening, and generalization of the DBT psychosocial skills: core mindfulness skills, distress tolerance, emotional regulation, and interpersonal effectiveness. Even when therapy-destructive behaviors are occurring, the best strategy at times is to ignore them and focus resolutely no matter what on teaching the skills in the module at hand; this is almost always the strategy employed with the less serious therapy-interfering behaviors. Active practice and use of behavioral skills are extremely difficult for borderline individuals since these require them to move out of their active-passivity pattern. Thus, if passive behavior is followed either by a group leader's shifting attention to another member (in a group context) or by a discussion of how the client is feeling or why she doesn't want to participate, this risks reinforcing the very behavior (passivity) that skills training is intended to reduce. At times, trainers can simply drag clients through difficult moments in skills training; such an approach, however, requires that the trainers be very sure of their behavioral assessments. The key point is that such an approach should be strategic rather than simply insensitive.

Therapy-Interfering Behaviors

Behaviors that interfere with therapy, but do not destroy it, are not ordinarily addressed systematically in skills training. This decision is based primarily on the fact that if therapy-interfering behaviors were a high priority target, trainers might never get around to the designated skills training. Skills training does not address the therapy process itself, except as the process is an avenue for teaching and practicing the skills being taught. Unless they threaten to destroy the therapy altogether or offer a particularly good opportunity for practicing the skills currently being taught, therapy-interfering behaviors are generally ignored. At most, these behaviors are commented on in a way that communicates the desirability of change, while at the same time letting the client know that very little time can be devoted to problems unrelated to the skills being taught. Thus, mood-dependent passivity, restlessness, pacing around the room, doodling, sitting in odd positions, attempts to discuss the week's crisis, oversensitivity to criticism, or anger at other clients will be ignored at times. The client is treated (ingeniously, at times) as if she is not engaging in the dysfunctional behaviors.

At other times, a skills trainer may instruct or urge such a client to try to apply her behavioral skills to the problem at hand. For example, a client who gets angry and threatens to leave may be instructed to try to practice her distress tolerance skills, or her anger management skills. A client who is withdrawn, dissociating, or overactive, may be urged to practice her mindfulness (attending to the activity of the moment) skills. The key point here is that if skills trainers allow skills training sessions to become focused on therapy process or clients' life crises, including suicidal behaviors and quality-of-life-interfering behaviors, then training in skills will be forfeited.

As I have discussed in Chapter 3 of this manual, there is a 15-minute wind-down period at the end of each skills training session. This time is an appropriate time to observe therapy-interfering behaviors — or, even more importantly, improvement in previous interfering behaviors. As long as everyone gets a chance to voice an observation, this time can be used as therapy process time. One of the advantages of an observing wind-down is that it provides a time and place for discussing behaviors that are interfering with therapy. (Cautions about this procedure are also discussed in Chapter 3.)

Skills Training Targets and Diary Cards

Like individual therapists, skills training therapists need to know about clients' behavioral progress (or lack of it) during the week between sessions. Several information-gathering approaches are used. First, on the back of the diary cards (Figure 4.1; see Chapter 6 of the text for a description of diary cards) are listed a number of the most important skills taught in the skills training segment of the therapy. Next to each skill is a space for recording whether or not the client actually practiced the skill during the week. The card is brought to skills

training sessions each week. In addition, each skills training module has its own set of diary sheets; clients are given these as the need arises. The beginning of each skills training session is devoted to a individual review with each client of her efforts at practicing skills during the previous week. If the card is not brought in, or if the client reports no practice effort or skill application, then this is viewed as a problem in self-management and is analyzed and discussed as such. The problem should be framed in such a way that whatever skills are currently being taught can be applied.

Behavioral Targets during Phone Calls

In standard DBT, clients are told at the beginning of treatment that the only phone calls generally allowed to or from skills training therapists are to give or obtain information that cannot wait (e.g., to let a skills trainer know that a client is going to miss the next session). Calls to resolve interpersonal conflicts of such magnitude that the client does not feel she can come to another session if the conflict is not resolved before the next session are also appropriate. The reason for this limitation is that when skills training is conducted in groups (as in our program), skills trainers can be overwhelmed with calls if they are willing to accept calls from all group members. In addition, the focus of a group leader on the individual as part of a group can be a difficult context to break, especially when an unexpected phone call requires an immediate shifting of context. Thus, the rationale is based on observing one's limits as a group therapist.

Skills Training Procedures

During skills training, and more generally throughout DBT, therapists must insist at every opportunity that the clients actively engage in the acquisition and practice of skills needed to cope with life as it is. In other words, they must directly, forcefully, and repeatedly challenge borderline individuals' passive problem-solving style. The procedures described below are applied by every DBT therapist across all modes of treatment where appropriate. They are applied in a formal way in the structured skills training modules.

There are three types of skills training procedures: (1) skill acquisition (e.g., instructions, modeling), (2) skill strengthening (e.g., behavioral rehearsal, feedback), and (3) skill generalization (e.g., homework assignments, discussion of similarities and differences in situations). In skill acquisition, a therapist is teaching new behaviors. In skill strengthening and generalization the therapist is trying both to fine-tune skilled behaviors and to increase

Date	Alcohol		Over-the-Counter Medications		Prescription Medications		Street/ Illicit Drugs		Suicidal Ideation (0-5)	Misery (0-5)	Self-Harm					Used Skills (0-7)*
	#	Specify	#	Specify	#	Specify	#	Specify			Urges (0-5)	Action Yes/No				
Mon																
Tue																
Wed																
Thu																
Fri																
Sat																
Sun																

*
0 = Not thought about or used	3 = Tried, but couldn't use them	6 = Didn't try, used them, they didn't help
1 = Thought about, not used, didn't want to	4 = Tried, could do them but they didn't help	7 = Didn't try, used them, helped
2 = Thought about, not used, wanted to	5 = Tried, could use them, helped	

SKILLS DIARY CARD   INSTRUCTIONS: Circle the days you worked on each skill.

1. Wise mind	Mon	Tues	Wed	Thu	Fri	Sat	Sun
2. Observe: just notice	Mon	Tues	Wed	Thu	Fri	Sat	Sun
3. Describe: put words on	Mon	Tues	Wed	Thu	Fri	Sat	Sun
4. Nonjudgmental stance	Mon	Tues	Wed	Thu	Fri	Sat	Sun
5. One-mindfully: in-the-moment	Mon	Tues	Wed	Thu	Fri	Sat	Sun
6. Effectiveness: focus on what works	Mon	Tues	Wed	Thu	Fri	Sat	Sun
7. Objective effectiveness: DEAR MAN	Mon	Tues	Wed	Thu	Fri	Sat	Sun
8. Relationship effectiveness: GIVE	Mon	Tues	Wed	Thu	Fri	Sat	Sun
9. Self-respect effectiveness: FAST	Mon	Tues	Wed	Thu	Fri	Sat	Sun
10. Reduce vulnerability: PLEASE	Mon	Tues	Wed	Thu	Fri	Sat	Sun
11. Build MASTERy	Mon	Tues	Wed	Thu	Fri	Sat	Sun
12. Build positive experiences	Mon	Tues	Wed	Thu	Fri	Sat	Sun
13. Opposite-to-emotion action	Mon	Tues	Wed	Thu	Fri	Sat	Sun
14. Distract	Mon	Tues	Wed	Thu	Fri	Sat	Sun
15. Self-soothe	Mon	Tues	Wed	Thu	Fri	Sat	Sun
16. Improve the moment	Mon	Tues	Wed	Thu	Fri	Sat	Sun
17. Pros and cons	Mon	Tues	Wed	Thu	Fri	Sat	Sun
18. Radical acceptance	Mon	Tues	Wed	Thu	Fri	Sat	Sun

FIGURE 4.1. Front (top) and back (bottom) of a DBT diary card. The entire back half of the card is used in skills training sessions; the front half is used in individual therapy except for the last column ("Used Skills"), which is also employed in skills training.

the probability that the person will use the skilled behaviors already in her repertoire in relevant situations. Skill strengthening and skill generalization, in turn, require the application of contingency procedures, exposure, and/or cognitive modification. That is, once the therapist is sure that a particular response pattern is within the client's current repertoire, then other procedures are applied to increase the client's effective behaviors in everyday life. It is this emphasis on active, self-conscious teaching, typical of behavioral and cognitive therapies, that differentiates DBT from many psychodynamic approaches to treating borderline clients. Some skills training procedures, however, are virtually identical to those used in supportive psychotherapy. The targets of skills training are determined by the parameters of DBT; the emphasis on certain skills over others is determined by behavioral analysis in each individual case.

Orienting and Committing to Skills Training: Task Overview

Orienting is a skills trainer's chief means of selling the new behaviors as worth learning and DBT procedures as likely to work. Skills training can only be accomplished if a person actively collaborates with the treatment program. Some clients both have skill deficits and are fearful about acquiring the new skills. It can be useful to point out here that learning a new skill does not mean actually having to use the skill. That is, a person can acquire a skill and then choose in each situation whether to use it or not. Sometimes clients do not want to learn new skills because they feel hopeless that anything will really help. I find it useful to point out that the skills I am teaching have helped either me or others that I know. However, a skills trainer cannot prove ahead of time that particular skills will actually help a given individual.

Before teaching any new skill, the trainer should give an overall rationale (or draw it in Socratic fashion from the client) for why the particular skill or set of skills might be useful. At times this may only require a comment or two; at other times it may require extensive discussion. At some point the skills trainer should also explain the rationale for his or her methods of teaching— that is, a rationale for the DBT skills training procedures. The most important point to make here, and to repeat as often as needed, is that learning new skills requires practice, practice, practice. Equally importantly, practice has to occur in situations where the skills are needed. If these points do not get through to a client, there is not much hope that she will actually learn anything new.

Skill Acquisition

Skill acquisition procedures are concerned with remediating skill deficits. DBT does not assume that all, or even most, of a borderline person's problems are motivational in nature. Instead, the bias is toward assessing the extent of the person's abilities in a particular area; skill acquisition procedures are then used if skill deficits exist. At times, in lieu of other means of assessment, the therapist employs skill acquisition procedures and then observes any consequent change in behavior.

A Note on Assessing Abilities

It can be very difficult with borderline clients to know whether they are incapable of doing something or are capable but emotionally inhibited or constrained by environmental factors. Although this is a complex assessment question with any client population, it can be particularly hard with borderline individuals because of their inability to analyze their own behavior and abilities. For example, they often confuse being afraid of doing something with not being *able* to do it. In addition, there are often powerful contingencies mitigating against their admitting having any behavioral capabilities. (I have reviewed many of these in Chapter 10 in the text.) Clients may say that they do not know how they feel or what they think, or that they can't find words, when in reality they are afraid of expressing the thoughts and feelings. As many of them say, they often do not want to be vulnerable. Some clients have been taught by their families and therapists to view all of their problems as motivationally based, and have either bought that story entirely (and thus believe they can do anything, but just do not want to) or have rebelled completely (and thus never entertain the possibility that motivational factors might be as important as ability-related factors). These therapy dilemmas are discussed more fully in the next chapter.

Some therapists respond to clients' statements that they can't do anything with an equally polarized statement that they can if only they want to. Failing to behave skillfully, and claiming not to know how to behave differently, are viewed as resistant (or at least as determined by motives outside awareness). Giving advice, coaching, making suggestions, or otherwise teaching new behaviors is seen as encouraging dependency and need gratification that gets in the way of "real" therapy. Other therapists, of course, fall into the trap of believing that clients can hardly do anything. At times they even go so far as to believe that the clients are incapable of learning new, more skillful behaviors. Acceptance, nurturance, and environmental intervention compromise the armamentarium of these therapists. Not surprisingly, when these two orientations coexist within a client's treatment team, conflict and "staff splitting" often arise. A dialectical approach would suggest looking for the synthesis, as I discussed more fully in Chapter 13 of the text.

To assess whether a behavioral pattern is within a client's repertoire, the skills trainer has to figure out a way to create ideal circumstances for her to produce the behavior. For interpersonal behaviors, an approximation to this is role playing during the skills training session — or, if the client refuses, asking her to indicate what she would say in a particular situation. Alternatively, one client can be asked to coach another during a role play. I am frequently amazed to find that individuals who appear very interpersonally skilled cannot put together reasonable responses in certain role-play situations, whereas individuals who seem passive, meek and unskilled are quite capable of responding skillfully if the role play can be made comfortable enough. In analyzing distress tolerance, the trainer can ask what techniques the client uses or thinks helpful in tolerating difficult or stressful situations. Emotion regulation can sometimes be assessed by interrupting an exchange and asking the client to see whether she can change her emotional state. Self-management and mindfulness skills can be analyzed by observing the client's behavior in sessions, especially when she is not the focus of attention, and questioning her about her day-to-day behavior.

If the client produces a behavior, the skills trainer knows she has it in her repertoire. However, if she does not, the trainer cannot be sure; as in statistics, there is no way to test the null hypothesis. When in doubt, it is usually safer to proceed with skill acquisition procedures, just in case. Generally, there is no harm in doing so and most of the procedures also affect other factors related to skilled behavior. For example, both instructions and modeling (the principal skill acquisition procedures; see below) may work also because they give the individual "permission" to behave, and thus reduce inhibitions, rather than because they add to the individual's behavioral repertoire.

Instructions

Instructions are verbal descriptions of the response components to be learned. They can vary from general guidelines ("When restructuring your thinking, be sure to check out the probability that the dire consequences will occur," "Think reinforcement") to very specific suggestions as to what the client should do ("The minute an urge hits, go get an ice cube and hold it in your hand for 10 minutes") or think ("Keep saying over and over to yourself, 'I can do it' "). Especially in a group setting, they can be presented in a lecture format with a black-

board as an aid. Instructions can be suggested as hypotheses to be considered, can be set forth as thesis and antithesis to be synthesized, or can be drawn out in a Socratic method of discourse. In all cases, a therapist must be careful not to oversimplify the ease of behaving effectively or of learning the skill. The skills training hand-outs in the back of this book provide written instructions.

Modeling

Modeling can be provided by therapists, other clients, other people in a client's environment, audiotapes, videotapes, films, or printed material. Any procedure that provides the client with examples of appropriate alternative responses is a form of modeling. The advantage of a skills trainer's providing the modeling is that the situation and materials can be tailored to fit a particular client's needs.

There are a number of ways to model skilled behavior. In-session role playing (with the skills trainer as a participant) can be used to demonstrate appropriate interpersonal behavior. When events between a trainer and the client arise that are similar to events the client encounters in her natural environment, the trainer can model handling such situations in effective ways. The skills trainer can also use self-talk (speaking aloud) to model coping self-statements, self-instructions, or restructuring of problematic expectations and beliefs. For example, the trainer may say, "OK, here's what I would say to myself: 'I'm overwhelmed. What's the first thing I do when overwhelmed? Break down the situation into steps and make a list. Do the first thing on the list.' " Telling stories, relating historical events, or providing allegorical examples (see Chapter 7 of the text) can often be useful in demonstrating alternative life strategies. Finally, self-disclosure can be used to model adaptive behavior, especially if a skills trainer has encountered problems in living similar to those a client is currently encountering. This tactic is discussed at length in Chapter 12 of the text, and careful attention to the guidelines listed there is recommended.

All of the modeling techniques describes above, of course, can also be used in a group context by members in modeling for one another. The ideal is for one group member to demonstrate in front of the whole group how to handle a situation skillfully. The more comfortable group members are with one another and with the group leader, the easier it is to induce them to act as models. Humor and flattery can be great aids here.

In addition to in-session modeling, it can be useful to have clients observe the behavior and responses of competent people in their own environment. The behaviors that they observe can then be discussed in sessions and practiced by everyone. The skills training hand-outs provide models of how to use specific skills. Biographies, autobiographies, and novels about people who have coped with similar problems provide new ideas as well. It is always important to discuss with the clients any behaviors modeled by the skills trainers or other clients, or presented as models outside of therapy, to be sure that the client is observing the relevant responses.

Skill Strengthening

Once skilled behavior has been acquired, skill strengthening is used to shape, refine, and increase the likelihood of their use. Without reinforced practice, a skill cannot be learned; this point cannot be emphasized too much, since skill practice is effortful behavior and directly counteracts borderline individuals' tendencies to employ a passive behavior style.

Behavioral Rehearsal

Behavioral rehearsal is any procedure in which a client practices responses to be learned. This can be done in interactions with therapists or other clients, and in simulated or *in vivo* situations. Any skilled behaviors—verbal sequences, nonverbal actions, patterns of thinking or cognitive problem solving, and some components of physiological and emotional responses—can, in principle, be practiced.

Practice can be either overt or covert. Various forms of overt behavioral rehearsal are possible. For example, in a group context, group members may role-play (together or with the leaders) problematic situations, so that each member can practice responding appropriately. To learn to control physiological responses, clients may practice relaxing during a session. In learning cognitive skills, each client may be asked to verbalize effective self-statements. In the specific case of cognitive restructuring, clients may be asked to first examine and verbalize any dysfunctional beliefs, rules, or possible expectancies elicited by the problem situation, and then to restructure these beliefs by generating more useful coping statements, rules, or the like. In group sessions, they can do this in writing (on handouts provided for this purpose) and then share what they have written with the group. Covert response practice—that is, practicing the requisite response in imagination—may also be an effective form of skill strengthening. It may be more effective than overt methods for teaching more complex cognitive skills, and it is also useful when a client refuses to engage in overt rehearsal. Clients can be asked to practice emotion regulation; generally, however, "emotional behavior" cannot be practiced directly. That is, clients cannot practice getting angry, feeling sad, or ex-periencing joy. Instead, they have to practice specific components of emotions (changing facial expressions, generating thoughts that elicit or inhibit emotions, changing muscle tension, etc.). In my experience, borderline individuals rarely like behavioral rehearsal, especially when it is done in front of others. Thus, a fair amount of cajoling and shaping is needed. If a client won't role-play an interpersonal situation, for example, a skills trainer can try talking her through a dialogue ("Then what could you say?"), or can try practicing just part of a new skill so that the client is not overwhelmed. The essence of the message here, though, is that in order to *be* different, people must practice *acting* differently. Some therapists do not like behavioral rehearsal either, especially when it requires them to role-play with the clients. For therapists who feel shy or uncomfortable, the best solution is for them to practice role playing with members of the supervision/consultation team. At other times, therapists resist role playing because they do not want to push rehearsal on clients. These therapists may not be aware of the wealth of data indicating that behavioral rehearsal is related to therapeutic improvement (e.g., Linehan, Goldfried, & Goldfried, 1979).

Response Reinforcement

Therapist reinforcement is one of the most powerful mean of shaping and strengthening skilled behavior in borderline and suicidal individuals. Frequently, such persons have lived in environments that overuse punishment. They often expect negative, punishing feedback from the world in general and their therapists in particular, and apply self-punishing strategies almost exclusively in trying to shape their own behavior. Over the long run, skill reinforcement by therapists can modify the clients' self-image in a positive manner, increase their use of skilled behavior, and enhance their sense that they can control positive outcomes in their lives. One of the benefits of group therapy over individual therapy is that when a group leader actively and obviously reinforces a skilled behavior in one group member, the same behavior among all other group members (if they are attending) is vicariously reinforced. In other words, this provides "more bang for the buck." Moreover, group therapy can be very powerful when group members become adept at reinforcing skilled behaviors in one another.

The techniques of providing appropriate reinforcement are discussed extensively in Chapter 10 of the text. Those principles are very important and should be reviewed thoroughly. Here, however, it is important to point out that skills trainers have to stay alert and notice client behaviors that represent improvement, even if these make the trainers rather uncomfortable. Teaching clients interpersonal skills to use with their parents, and then punishing or ignoring those same skills when used in a training session, for example, is not therapeutic. Encouraging clients to think for themselves, but then punishing or ignoring them when they disagree with a trainer, is not therapeutic. Stressing that "not fitting in" in all circumstances is not a disaster and that distress can be tolerated, and then not tolerating clients when they do not fit comfortably into a trainer's schedule or preconceived notions of how borderline individuals act, is not therapeutic.

Feedback and Coaching

Response feedback is the provision of information to clients about their performance. Feedback should pertain to performance, not to the motives presumably leading to the performance. This point is very important. One of the unfortunate factors in the lives of many borderline individuals is that people rarely give them feedback about their behavior that is uncontaminated with interpretations about their presumed motives and intent. When the presumed motives do not fit, the individuals often discount or are distracted from the valuable feedback they may be getting about their behavior. Feedback should be behaviorally specific; that is, a skills trainer should tell the client exactly what she is doing that seems to indicate either continuing problems or improvement. Telling clients that they are manipulating, expressing a need to control, overreacting, clinging, or acting out is simply not helpful if there are not clear behavioral referents for the terms. This is, of course, especially true when a trainer has pin-pointed a problem behavior correctly but is making inaccurate motivational inferences. Many arguments between clients and therapists arise out of just this inaccuracy. The role and use of interpretation in DBT are discussed extensively in Chapter 9 of the text.

A skills trainer must attend closely to a client's behavior (within sessions or self-reported) and select those responses on which to give feedback. At the beginning of training, the client may do little that appears competent; the trainer is usually well advised at this point to give feedback on a limited number of response components, even though other deficits could be commented upon. Feedback on more may lead to stimulus overload and/or discouragement about the rate of progress. A response shaping paradigm (discussed in Chapter 10 of the text) should be used, with feedback, coaching, and reinforcement designed to encourage successive approximations to the goal of effective performance.

Borderline individuals often desperately want feedback about their behavior, but at the same time are sensitive to negative feedback. The solution here is to surround negative feedback with positive feedback. Treating clients as too fragile to deal with negative feedback does them no favor. An important part of feedback is giving clients information about the effects of their behavior on their therapists; this is discussed more extensively in Chapter 12 of the text.

Coaching is combining feedback with instructions. It is telling the client how a response is discrepant from the criterion of skilled performance and how it might be improved. Clinical practice suggests that the "permission" to behave in certain ways that is implicit in coaching may sometimes be all that is needed to accomplish changes in behavior.

Skill Generalization

DBT does not assume that skills learned in therapy will necessarily generalize to situations in everyday life outside of therapy. Therefore, it is very important that skills trainers actively encourage this transfer of skills. Although skill generalization is the primary responsibility of the primary or individual psychotherapist (because of time limitations in skills training therapy), there are a number of specific procedures that skills trainers can use as well.

Between-Session Consultation

If they are unable to apply new skills in their natural environment, clients should be encouraged to get consultation from their individual psychotherapists and from one another between sessions. Skills trainers can give these individuals lessons on how to provide appropriate coaching. On inpatient and day treatment units, clients can be encouraged to seek assistance from staff members when they are having difficulty. Another technique, developed by Charles Swenson at Cornell Medical Center/New York Hospital at White Plains and mentioned in Chapter 2 of this manual, is to provide a unit behavioral consultant with regular office hours. The consultant's task is to help clients apply their new skills to everyday life.

Review of Session Tapes

If possible, skills training sessions should be videotaped. The videotapes can then be reviewed by client between sessions if there is a room available where they can come and watch tapes. There are several reasons for the tape monitoring strategy. First, because of substance abuse prior to sessions, high emotional arousal during sessions, dissociation or other concentration difficulties accompanying depression and anxiety, clients are often unable to attend to much of what transpires during a skills training session. Thus, the patients may improve their retention of material offered during the session by viewing the videotape. Second, a client may gain important insights from viewing herself and her interactions with others. Such insights often help the client understand and improve her own interpersonal skills. Third, many clients report that coming in to watch a skills training tape can be very helpful when they are feeling overwhelmed, panicked, or unable to cope between sessions. Simply watching a tape, especially if they can find one of a session where a needed skill was taught, has an effect similar to that of having an additional session. Skills trainers should encourage, but not require or demand, use of the tapes for these purposes.

In Vivo *Behavioral Rehearsal Assignments*

In structured skills training, homework assignments are keyed to the specific behavioral skills currently being taught. It is advantageous if a skills trainer or a client can also get the client's individual psychotherapist to use some of the homework assignments and accompanying forms throughout therapy, or on an as-needed basis. This is always done in standard DBT. For example, one of the structured homework forms focuses on identifying and labeling emotions and takes the client through a series of steps to help her clarify what she is feeling. The individual therapist may suggest that the client use this form whenever she is confused or overwhelmed by emotions. At the back of this manual are a number of homework assignment sheets, covering each of the DBT behavioral skills. There is no reason, of course, why skills trainers and individual therapists cannot revise these forms to fit either their clients' or their own personal preferences and needs.

Creating an Environment That Reinforces Skilled Behavior

As I discuss in Chapter 3 of the text, borderline individuals tend to have a passive style of personal regulation. On the continuum whose poles are internal self-regulation and external environmental regulation, they are near the environmental pole. Many therapists seem to believe that the self-regulation pole of the continuum is inherently better or more mature, and spend a fair amount of therapy time trying to make borderline individuals more self-regulated. Although DBT does not suggest the converse—that environmental regulation styles are preferable—it does suggest that going with the clients' strength is likely to be easier and more beneficial in the long run. Thus, once behavioral skills are in place, clients should be taught how to maximize the tendency of their natural environments to reinforce skilled over unskilled behaviors. This may include teaching them how to create structure, how to make public instead of private commitments, how to find communities and lifestyles that support their new behaviors, and how to elicit reinforcement from others for skilled rather than unskilled behaviors. This is not to say that clients should not be

taught self-regulation skills; rather, the types of self-regulation skills taught should be keyed to their strengths. Written self-monitoring with a prepared diary form, for example, is preferable over trying to observe behavior each day and make a mental note of it. Keeping alcohol out of the house is preferable to trying a self-talk strategy to inhibit getting out the bottle.

A final point needs to be made here. Sometimes clients' newly learned skills do not generalize because out in the real world they punish their own behavior. This is usually because their behavioral expectations for themselves are so high that they simply never reach the criterion for reinforcement. This pattern must change if generalization and progress are to occur. Problems with self-reinforcement and self-punishment are discussed more extensively in Chapters 3, 8, and 10 of the text; the behavioral validation strategies described in Chapter 8 should be used in skills training as well. I discuss these topics further in the skills module content chapters of this manual (7–10).

Family and Couples Sessions. One way to maximize generalization is to have individuals from the client's social community come to sessions. Usually, these will be members of the clients' families or their spouses or partners. Perry Hoffman, of Cornell Medical Center/New York Hospital at White Plains has developed a form of family therapy in which borderline clients and members of their families are brought together as a group. The same skills modules used with the borderline clients without their families present are then retaught with their families present. Thus, all members of the family are learning the same sets of skills. Since the borderline clients are usually a lesson or two ahead of their families, they can assist in teaching family members the DBT behavioral skills. Family members of borderline clients have been very receptive to this type of therapy.

Principles of Fading. At the beginning of skills training, the therapist models, instructs, reinforces, gives feedback, and coaches the client for using skills both within the therapy sessions and in her natural environment. If skillful behavior in the everyday environment is to become independent of the influence of the therapist, however, then the therapist must gradually fade out his or her use of these procedures, particularly instructions and reinforcement. The goal here is to fade skills training procedures to an intermittent schedule, such that the therapist is providing less frequent instructions and coaching than the client can provide for herself, and less modeling, feedback, and reinforcement than the client is obtaining from her natural environment.

5

Application of Other Strategies and Procedures to Psychosocial Skills Training

The major strategies and procedures in DBT are discussed in detail in the text accompanying this manual. This chapter is along the lines of "OK, if you know all that, here's what else to think about when you apply it to skills training especially in a group setting." The text provides the rationale, theory, and caveats for each set of strategies and procedures; skills trainers need to know these in order to respond flexibly to new problems that arise. This chapter addresses some of the problems that may arise specifically in skills training and some of the modifications of strategies and procedures I have found useful, particularly in a group context.

Dialectical Strategies

As noted in the Chapter 7 of the text, the dialectical focus in DBT occurs at two levels of therapeutic behavior. At the first level, a therapist must be alert to the dialectical balance occurring within the treatment environment. In a group setting, each group member, (including each leader) is in a constant state of dialectical tension at many levels and in many directions. The first set of tensions consists of the tensions between each individual member and the group as a whole. From this perspective, the group has an identity of its own, and each member can react to the group as a whole. Thus, for example, a member may be acting in dialectical tension with group norms, group beliefs or attitudes, or group "personality." In addition, insofar as the identity of the group as a whole is both the sum of and more than its

parts, the identity of each individual in the group is in some aspect defined by her relationship to the group. Because both the identity of the group and the identity of each individual change over the year, identification of members with the group and the struggles that evolve with this identity provide a dialectical tension that can be harnessed for the sake of therapeutic progress.

A second set of tensions consists of those between each individual pair within the group—tensions that can become active at any moment when two group members interact. A drawback of allowing members to interact with one another outside of the group is that relationships between members can develop outside of the public arena of the group. Thus, the dialectical tensions between one member and another will often not be apparent to the leaders or other group members. Overlaying and interfacing with these two levels, so to speak, is a third set of dialectical tensions between each individual and her unique environment—a context bought into the treatment situation via long term memory.

The group leaders must be aware of the multiple tensions impinging on a skills training session at any given time. Maintaining a therapeutic balance and moving the balance toward reconciliation and growth are the tasks of the therapists. It is essential here that each therapist remember that he or she is also a group member and thus is also in dialectical tension with the group as a whole, with the other leader, and with each individual member.

Clearly, the dialectical framework that is necessary

here is that of a dynamic, open system. The system includes not only those present but also all external influences that are brought into group sessions via long-term memory and established behavioral patterns. This framework will help the group leaders avoid the mistake of always interpreting members' behavior from the point of view of a closed system. The closed-system perspective assumes that all responses are a direct reaction to events within sessions. It is far more common, however, for a group activity or event to precipitate the remembering of events that have occurred outside of sessions. Borderline clients are quite unable to put aside or stop cognitive processing of very stressful events, or ruminating, and focus on one thing in the moment. It is also a mistake, on the other hand, for the leaders never to attribute client behavior to in-session events. It is this dialectical tension between and among influential events that the leaders must be attuned to.

The second level of dialectical focus is on teaching and modeling dialectical thinking as a replacement for dichotomous, either–or, black-and-white thinking. Techniques such as entering the paradox, storytelling and other uses of metaphor, extending, playing the devil's advocate, activating "wise mind," making lemonade out of lemons, dialectical assessment, and allowing natural change are described in Chapter 7 of the text and are applicable to skills training. (I discuss specific applications of some of these techniques later.) The group setting, in particular, offers a rich environment for demonstrating the futility of approaching problem solving with a "right versus wrong" cognitive set. No matter how brilliant a solution to a particular problem may be, it is always possible for another group member or for the member with the problem to come up with another strategy that may be equally effective. And every problem solution has its own set of limitations; that is, there is always "another side of the story." It is extremely important that the group leaders not get into a battle of trying to prove that the skills being taught are the only right way to handle every situation, or even any particular situation. Although the skills may be very effective for some purposes, they are not more "right" than other approaches. Thus, the leaders' task is to ask this question repeatedly: "How can we all be right, and how can we test the effectiveness of our strategies?"

A group also offers a unique opportunity to observe the process of change and development. It can be very difficult to see change and development in oneself; it is often easier to see it in another. The leaders' task here is to comment on the evolutionary process of both the group as a whole and of each individual, and to encourage members to begin observing the same phenomenon.

Typical Dialectics

Willingness versus Willfulness

The tension between "willingness" and "willfulness" is an important one in treating borderline clients. Although I discuss it much more fully in Chapter 10 of this manual, the essential tension is between responding to a situation in terms of what the situation needs (willingness) and responding in a way that resists what a situation needs or responding in terms of one's own needs rather than those of the situation (willfulness). Thus, willfulness encompasses both trying to "fix" the situation and sitting passively on one's hands, refusing to respond at all.

There are many forms of this tension in conducting skills training with borderline clients. A key one arises in a group context when the leaders are interacting with one member or the group as a whole, and the member or group is withdrawing and refusing to interact. The tension is between attempting to influence the member or group and allowing oneself to be influenced by the member or group. The essential question, framed somewhat more directly, is how far the leaders should push and how far the group member or group as a whole should resist. Use of the terms "willfulness" and "willingness" can be quite helpful in this dilemma. I have found myself on many occasions discussing with a client who is being willful—I, she, or both of us. Of course, the answer to the question revolves around what is needed in the situation, and it is at this point that skill becomes important. It is also, however, a matter of perspective or dialectical focus. The group leaders must keep in mind the member's or group's needs at the moment and in the long term, or current comfort versus future gain, and balance these respective goals. If this balance is missed, then the leaders are in danger of being willful. It is all too easy to get into a power struggle with group members, in which the needs of the leaders to make progress, to feel effective, or to create a more comfortable atmosphere come into conflict with the needs of the members.

The problem of willfulness versus willingness is nowhere more apparent than when a therapist is juggling the needs of an individual group member and those of the group as a whole. This most commonly occurs when one member is refusing to interact, is hostile, or otherwise is behaving in a way that influences the mood, comfort, and progress of the entire group. In my experience, such a threat to the group's good can bring out in a therapist the tendency to be willful. Generally, the tension here is between two types of willfulness. On the one hand, a therapist can be willful by actively controlling, and attacking the errant member or her behavior. Because group members are singularly unskilled at coping with negative affect, when one member creates conflict other group members withdraw. As the mood of the group becomes increasingly tense or hopeless, the therapist naturally wants to turn it around; thus, the attempt to control the member initiating the conflict ensues. In contrast the therapist can be equally willful by ignoring the conflict and tense mood and responding in a passive way. Passivity in this case actually masquerades as activity, since ignoring the tension is generally manifested by the therapist's continuing to push and escalate the conflict.

The synthesis of willfulness on each side is willingness. Willingness is a response that balances the needs of the individual versus the needs of the group as a whole, and the needs of the moment versus the long-term benefits for the group. Unfortunately, no manual can pinpoint where this balance is in the individual case.

"Good Guy versus Bad Guy"

In a group setting, keeping group members working together collaboratively is often very hard work for the leaders. Variations in individual members' moods when they arrive for a session, as well as reactions to in-session events, can have a tremendous effect on any given individual's willingness to work collaboratively during a particular group meeting. It is not untypical that an entire group may be "out of the mood," so to speak, for working at a particular meeting. When this happens, the leaders must continue to interact with the group members in an attempt to get them working collaboratively again. However, this attempt to interact with the members is often viewed by the members as "pushing," and the leader doing the work is (usually, the primary group leader) viewed as the "bad guy" by the group members. At this point it is often helpful for the coleader to validate the group members' experience. As they are pushed by the primary leader, they often not only retreat but become more rigid in their refusal to interact. Validation from the coleader can reduce the negative affect and enhance their ability to work. When this occurs, however, the coleader may then be viewed as the "good guy." Thus the dialectical tension builds between the coleaders. This scenario is closely related to the psychodynamic concept of "splitting."

The danger is that the leaders will allow themselves to become "split," so to speak, acting as independent units rather than a cohesive whole. This is most likely to happen if either of the leaders begins to see his or her position as "right" and the other leader's position as "wrong." Once this happens, the leaders pull away from one another and disturb the balance that might otherwise occur. This will not go unnoticed, because

group members watch the relationship between the leaders closely. I often refer to group skills training as a recreation of family dinners. Most members have many experiences of unresolved conflicts and battles occurring at family dinners. Group skills training is an opportunity for members to experience a wholeness in the resolution of conflict. The leaders' ability to contain the dialectic in their relationship—to stay united and whole, even as they take different roles—is essential for this learning. Of course, being the "good guy" can be quite comfortable and being the "bad guy" can be quite uncomfortable. Thus, it takes some skillfulness and personal feelings of security for the primary leader to take the role of the "bad guy." (I should be careful to note here that it is not always the primary leader who is the "bad guy." At times, either leader can take this role.)

Another dialectical tension that may build is that between the skills training leaders and the clients' individual psychotherapists. Here the skills trainers can either be the "good guys" or the "bad guys," and the individual therapists can play the corresponding role. In my experience, during the first year of DBT, the skills trainers are more often the "bad guys" and the individual therapists are the "good guys"; however, on occasion the roles are switched. In fact, this is one of the great assets of separating skills training from individual therapy in DBT: It allows a client to have a "bad guy" and a "good guy" simultaneously. Thus, the client is often able to tolerate staying in therapy more readily.

The function of the "good guy" is often to hold the client in therapy while she resolves her conflicts with the "bad guy." Most borderline individuals do not have the experience of staying in a painful relationship long enough to work a conflict out and then to experience the reinforcement of conflict resolution. DBT, therefore, offers perhaps a unique context in which this can be done. In a sense, a client always has a benign consultant to help her deal with her conflicts with the other therapist. The essential ingredient here, as should be obvious, is that whoever is the "good guy" must always be able to hold in mind the therapeutic relationships as a whole, rather than allowing them to resolve into "right versus wrong" and true "good guy versus bad guy." It is the therapists' ability to hold these relationships as a whole that will eventually allow their clients to learn to do the same. As the therapists model balance, clients will learn to balance themselves.

Content versus Process

As noted previously, process issues are not attended to systematically during group skills training except when negative process threatens to destroy the group. However, even when this threat emerges, it may be that borderline clients simply cannot process conflict in a group setting. (Even in individual skills training, if the relationship is intense, the skills trainer may not be able to resolve interpersonal issues promptly. Especially when the skills trainer is also the individual therapist, issues from individual psychotherapy sessions may spill over into the skills training). The tension that arises is between whether the group leaders should proceed with teaching content, even though members are passive, are hostile, don't want to learn, are angry at one another, or feel rejected, and whether the leaders should stop and discuss the conflicts and dissatisfactions and attend to the process in the group.

Attending to process is fraught with difficulties in the first year. In our clinic the group therapy program is a multiyear program; our experience is that borderline clients are not able to deal with group process before the second year of therapy. The first-year group wind-downs are the training ground for group process. More than a few minutes of process is often more than group members can handle. The danger here is that a conflict beginning in group sessions may not be resolved because members walk out or the sessions end. When this happens and the conflict is serious, the group leaders may need to spend considerable time talking with each member individually to help her work through the issues. Thus, if process is to be attended to, content may have to be dropped at least temporarily. On the other hand, if content alone is attended to without any attention to process, the group will break down eventually. Holding the balance between content and process, is essential.

In my experience, some group leaders do better with content and find it easy to ignore process, whereas other group leaders do well with process and find it easy to ignore content. It is rare that a group leader will find achieving this critical balance an easy task. Perhaps the key here is recognizing the pull of borderline individuals toward making every moment they are in comfortable. Their inability to put discomfort on a shelf and attend to a task poses a formidable obstacle to continuing with content when process issues are in the foreground. We have found it necessary, however, time and again to forge ahead. Forging ahead generally requires the therapists to ignore some of the process issues and respond as if group members are collaborating even when they are not. It is a delicate balance that can only be mastered with experience.

Following the Rules versus Reinforcing Assertiveness

As noted in Chapter 3 of this manual, DBT skills training has a number of rules. These rules are not unimportant, and some of them are unequivocal and unbendable. On the other hand, a primary target in DBT is teaching interpersonal skills, including the ability to assert oneself. A tension that arises over time, if skills trainers are doing their job well, is that between maintaining the rules (regardless of clients' assertions and requests to the contrary) and reinforcing clients' growing assertive skills by bending the rules when requested to in an appropriate manner. The ability to balance "giving in" and "not giving in" is essential. It is here that the trainers' attitude of compassionate flexibility must be balanced with unwavering centeredness (qualities discussed in Chapter 4 of the text).

What is required is clear thinking on the part of the skills trainers. Giving in for the sake of giving in is as rigid as holding to rules for the sake of holding on. The simple fact that a client requests that a rule be bent or broken in an appropriate manner, however, is not sufficient for reward. Clearly, appropriate requests are not always met with a gracious response in the real world. In fact, one of the key misconceptions of borderline individuals is that if they ask appropriately, the world will (or should) always give them what they need or want. Learning to deal with the fact that this does not always happen is essential for growth and is one of the goals of distress tolerance training (see Chapter 10 of this manual). On the other hand, the attempt to teach this fundamental lesson should not be confused with arbitrary refusals to make exceptions when the situation requires it. Once again, the notion of willingness can be viewed as the synthesis, and thus as the path for the therapists to follow.

Willingness, however, requires clarity on the skills' trainers' part. The clarity needed has to do with the ultimate goals of therapy for an individual member (or for the group, in a group setting) and the means of achieving the goals. The tension that most often exists is that between current comfort and learning to deal with discomfort. Therapists must straddle these two aims in coming to a decision about what is the most effective response to a client's assertive behavior.

The task is much easier, of course, if the skills trainers can see emerging client assertiveness as progress rather than as a threat. This is often not very comfortable, because life becomes much more difficult for the trainers when clients begin interacting as peers rather than as "patients." The "one up, one down" relationship that so often exists in therapy is threatened as the clients make progress. To the extent that the skills trainers can take delight in the clients' emerging abilities to outreason, outlogic, and outmaneuver them, therapy progress will be enhanced and not threatened. Essential here in a group context, of course, is respecting the other group members' point of view. It is also essential for the trainers to recognize when they are up against a brick wall and are not going to win their point anyway. At these times, the willingness to bend the rules and agree to a client's assertive request can sometimes radically change the nature of the therapeutic relationship.

The use of two leaders in conducting group treatment offers further avenues for setting up a dialectic, as noted earlier. In essence, each group leader's style can function as one element in the dialectical opposition. For example, a "good cop, bad cop" strategy, in which one leader focuses on content while the other focuses on process can be used. Or one leader can help the other leader and a group member synthesize a tension or conflict. While one leader presents one side of the whole, the other leader presents the contrasting side.

Specific Dialectical Strategies

Although therapists will use all of the dialectical strategies at one time or another, some are particularly useful in skills training. The first task in teaching core mindfulness skills (see Chapter 7 of this manual) is to familiarize clients with the concept of "wise mind." The strategy of activating "wise mind" should then be employed throughout skills training. When a client makes a statement representing an emotional or feeling state (e.g., "I feel fat or unlovable") as if the feeling state provides information about the empirical reality ("I am fat or unlovable"), it is effective at times simply to question the client: "I'm not interested in how you feel. I'm not interested in what you believe or think. I am interested in what you know to be true (in your 'wise mind'). What do you know to be true? What is true?" The dialectical tension here is between what the client feels to be true ("emotion mind") and what she thinks to be true ("reasonable mind"); the synthesis is what she knows to be true. The push toward "wise mind" can be easily abused, of course, especially when the therapist confuses "wise mind" with what the therapist believes to be the case. This can be particularly difficult when the therapist trusts the wisdom of his or her own knowledge or opinions. The value of therapeutic humility cannot be overstated. In DBT, one of the major functions of the supervision/consultation group is to provide a balance to the arrogance that can easily accompany the therapist's powerful position.

Almost any disaster or crisis is an opportunity to practice skills; this is an example of making lemonade out of lemons (i.e., finding the positives in a negative situation). As I have noted in Chapter 2 of this manual, conducting an open (rather than closed) group offers an opportunity to allow natural change, another dialectical strategy. Finally, therapists should be prepared to use story, myth, and parable to get across what they mean when teaching complex skills. In the case of mindful-

ness skills, there is often no other way to communicate the essence of the message.

Problem-Solving Strategies

Problem-solving strategies (discussed in detail in Chapter 9 of the text) are the backbone of the practice sharing component of skills training. In our model for group skills training, this comprises the first 50–60 minutes of every session. Problem-solving strategies are crucial in describing patterns over time, analyzing particular problematic situations and developing more effective coping strategies. The goal here is to get clients to begin using the problem solving strategies with one another and, of course, eventually with themselves.

Behavioral Analysis

In a group setting, the first step in practice sharing is for each group member to share with the group the particular skills she used (and their success or failure), as well as the situations she used them in during the previous week. (In an individual context, the client describes her skill usage during the week to her skills trainer.) Clients will inevitably present their situations and/or skill use in very general and vague terms at first. The first task of a skills trainer is to get a client to describe, step by step, the particular environmental and behavioral events leading up to the problem situation and to the successful or nonsuccessful attempt to use the skills. The skills trainer must lead the client through an exhaustive chain analysis of the problem. (How to do this, where to start and stop, and roadblocks to avoid are described in detail in Chapter 9 of the text.)

Obviously, providing such a description requires that a client be able to observe during the week. Often clients have great difficulty describing what happened because they are not astute observers; however, with repeated practice and repeated reinforcement over the weeks, their observation and description skills tend to improve. A minute description allows a trainer to assess whether a client in fact used the skills appropriately. If the client was successful, this description in a group setting models for other clients how they can use those same skills for similar problems. Thus, the leader should try briefly to elicit from other group members examples of either similar problems or similar skill usage to foster this generalization.

Often, however, a client has not used skills successfully: Either she couldn't apply the skills, or they didn't work when she did apply them. It is extremely important at this point to lead the client through a very detailed examination of just what did occur. This can be tortur--

ous because almost always (especially during the first several months of therapy) clients are fearful of skills trainers' (and, in a group setting, other members') judgments and are also judging themselves in very negative ways. Thus, they can be expected to be very inhibited.

Sometimes a client will jump right in with a notion of why a skill didn't work or why she couldn't apply it, without examining the actual events. These explanations are frequently pejorative and involve name calling (e.g., "I am just stupid"). Or a client may accept without question the premise that her situation is hopeless and skills will never help. Borderline individuals seem particularly unable to analyze objectively and calmly just what leads up to a particular problem, especially when the problem is their own behavior. Obviously, if they cannot conduct such an analysis, attempts to solve the problem are probably doomed from the start. Many are unable to see the critical role of environmental context in behavior and persist in viewing all behavior as a function of internal motives, needs, and the like. (It is, of course, essential that skills trainers not collude with this view.) Thus, the skills trainer's task here is to engage the client in a behavioral analysis; to model nonpejorative, nonjudgmental behavioral evaluations; and (in a group context) to get both the individual and the group engaged in the process so that the same skills can be used in other problem situations.

Almost all incidents of noncompliance with homework assignments (i.e., refusing or forgetting to practice skills) and of refusal or failure to engage in skills training activities should elicit an immediate movement into behavioral analysis with the client involved. The tendency of the client to offer simple solutions and answers must be counteracted. When a client reports that she did not do any homework practice, the first step is to get a precise definition of the behaviors missing. In eliciting this information, I focus on four variables: (1) whether the client thought about practicing; (2) whether the client felt motivated to practice; (3) whether the client attempted to practice some skill or problem-solving response; and (4) whether the response worked (i.e., made things better). For example, a client may have never thought about practicing the skills after leaving the session; may have thought about practicing but didn't want to practice, may have thought about it, and wanted to practice, but couldn't figure out how to do it; or forgot to do it; and so on. Such a behavioral description begins to highlight the variables that may be important influencing factors in noncompliance.

If a client reports not ever thinking about home practice, then the task is to analyze what factors are related to her not remembering (the problem to be solved). Usually, the first several times this reason for noncompliance is reported, I describe the processes of short-term and long-term memory. I then help the client analyze whether the problem was that the idea of doing practice simply never made it out of short-term into long-term memory or that once it was in long-term memory nothing ever evoked the memory to operate. Often, I find that practicing does not get into long-term memory because the client doesn't attend during the session when practice is discussed. If the problem is not one of memory but one of lack of motivation, then this is analyzed. The most important thing to remember here is to offer nonpejorative hypotheses and communicate to the client a nonjudgmental attitude; the client is usually judgmental enough. Hypotheses that are particularly worthy of exploration include hopelessness that the skills will do any good; hopelessness that the client can ever learn the skills; beliefs that she doesn't need the skills and already has them; and beliefs that she should have learned these skills earlier, and therefore, is inadequate or stupid for having to learn them now. Such beliefs probably lead to negative emotional reactions, which the client then flees from. It is very important here to communicate to clients that it is OK to have hopeless beliefs, and that the skills trainers will not feel invalidated if the clients do not have perfect trust in them. Although each of these beliefs may be perfectly reasonable (and should be validated), holding on to the beliefs is probably not useful, and thus cheerleading (see Chapter 8 in the text), cognitive modification (see Chapter 11 in the text), and solution analysis (see below) are in order.

Sometimes a client reports that she tried to use the skills she was supposed to practice but could not carry them out. For example, a client may enter an interpersonal situation with every intent of applying some of the interpersonal effectiveness skills learned previously, but she may get confused and forget what to say or how to respond to a particular remark by the other person. At other times, a client may report using the skill appropriately, except that it didn't work. Even the most skilled negotiator cannot always get what she wants; relaxation exercises, even when used correctly, do not always lead to reduction of anxiety and tension. In these instances, it is essential to get precise information about what happened. A client and a therapist may both be tempted is to skip this and decide that this particular skill is not useful for this particular client. Although this may be true, it may also be true that the client is not applying the skill in the correct way.

Insight (Interpretation) Strategies

The insight strategies will be used primarily during homework sharing and during the observation winddowns. During homework sharing, it is very important to look carefully for patterns in situational problems, as well as typical responses to such problems. Highlighting idiosyncratic patterns can be especially helpful in future behavioral analyses. As mentioned previously, it is very important for clients to use a variety of strategies in coping with problem situations and emotions. Skills trainers should comment on any rigid patterns that they see, as well as on effective patterns or skills that the clients use. Clients' observations and comments about their own or one another's skillful patterns should, of course, be observed and reinforced. It is essential to follow the guidelines provided in the insight section in Chapter 9 of the text. In a group context, comments about group members' behavior not only communicate to the individuals in question, but give information to all members about how they should evaluate and interpret their own behavior.

The observing wind-down at the end of each session is another opportunity to utilize insight strategies in a group setting. Here it is particularly useful for the group leaders to comment on patterns of group interactions and group changes that they have noticed. Such insights highlight and foster the growth of dialectical thinking.

Solution Analysis

To a large extent, skills training is a general case of solution analysis. Skills are presented as practical solutions to life's problems, and the potential effectiveness of various skills in particular situations is discussed during each meeting. Perhaps more than any other set of strategies, solution analysis utilizes the power of a group context. Each member should be encouraged to offer solution ideas to other group members and to help develop strategies to solve the problems described. For example, a member who is having trouble paying attention during group sessions and getting homework assignments into short-term memory can be helped to think of ways to attend more closely. The group as a whole can almost always be counted on to come up with many solutions to not remembering to practice during the week. Difficulties in selecting the right skill to use or in applying a skill in a particular situation are further opportunities for group solution analysis. Almost always, someone will already have solved the problem at hand for herself; thus, the group leaders should be especially careful in the solution analysis phase not to jump in with solutions before eliciting possible solutions from other group members. However, they should not be reluctant to offer a solution or a particular application of a skill, even if other group members have offered other ideas.

Didactic Strategies

The second half of each skills training session is primarily didactic; during this section the therapists are teaching new material, generally through lectures and discussions. It is this direct teaching that constitutes didactic strategies. As the skills are taught, it is critical to attempt to link each skill to its intended outcome. For example, in teaching relaxation, skills trainers should describe not only how relaxation works but when it works, why it works, and what it works for. It is also useful to discuss when it doesn't work, why it may not work, and how to make it work when it seems not to be working. The more trouble trainers can predict in advance, the better clients are likely to learn the skill.

It is particularly important to remember that immediate emotional relief is not the goal of every skill taught in DBT skills training. This distinction is often not grasped by clients. In fact, almost always when they say that something didn't work, they mean that it didn't make them feel better immediately. Thus, the relationship of skills to long-term goals versus short-term goals, and to long-term relief versus immediate relief has to be discussed over and over. It is particularly important not to be pulled into always trying to show how a skilled behavior will make a person feel better right away. First, it isn't usually true; second, even if it were true it is not necessarily beneficial.

Orienting Strategies

The necessity for orientation in psychotherapy comes mostly from the relationship of psychotherapy to other forms of structured learning tasks. Knowing exactly what the task is, what one's role is, and what one can expect from the other person facilitates learning enormously. I have discussed the principles of orienting clients to skills training in general, and to each specific module, in the preceding chapter. The thing to remember here, however, is that orientation is called for with each specific skill and with each homework assignment.

Commitment Strategies

As I say repeatedly throughout both this book and the text, getting the client to commit herself to therapy, to learning, and to changing her behavior is all-important in DBT. I have discussed in the preceding chapter the necessity of getting an overall commitment to therapy. In skills training, the client also needs to make a re-commitment to each treatment module, as well as a commitment every week to practice new skills between sessions.

Validation Strategies

The validation strategies (discussed in detail in Chapter 8 of the text) are absolutely essential to DBT. It was the necessity of combining validation with problem-solving strategies and other change procedures that first led me to develop a "new" version of cognitive–behavioral therapy. As in individual psychotherapy, validation strategies are used in every skills training session in DBT. They involve a nonjudgmental therapeutic attitude and a continual search for the essential validity of each clients' responses (and, in a group context, those of the group as a whole). In group settings, both the leaders and the group as a whole function as the opposing pole to the invalidating environments commonly experienced by borderline individuals.

The first general task in validating is to help clients observe and accurately describe their own emotions, thoughts, and overt behavior patterns. Much of DBT psychosocial skills training—in particular, mindfulness training—is aimed at just this. Second, skills trainers communicate empathy with clients' emotional tone, indicate understanding of (though not necessarily agreement with) their beliefs and expectancies, and/or make clear observations of their behavioral action patterns. In other words, the trainers observe and describe the clients' behavior accurately. Third, and most importantly, the trainers communicate that the clients' emotional responses, beliefs and expectancies, and overt behaviors are understandable and make sense in the context of their lives and the current moment. In each instance, the trainers look for the nugget of gold in the cup of sand—the validity within what may otherwise be a very dysfunctional response. This is the reverse of the invalidating environment's approach.

In both group and individual skills training, almost constant cheerleading is necessary. The skills trainers' biggest problem here will probably be maintaining the energy necessary to cajole, prod, sweet-talk, and cheer on the clients' very slow movement in adopting new, more skillful behaviors. The tensions between "I can't/I won't" and "You can/You must" can drain even the most energetic therapist. In a group context, each group leader must rely on the other to provide fresh energy when he or she is losing steam and to bail him or her out of a willful dialogue with members.

It is equally important in group skills training to elicit and reinforce clients' validation of one another. The ability to validate others is one of the skills taught in the interpersonal effectiveness module. Borderline individuals, although noteworthy in their ability to empathize with and validate one another, are also capable of highly judgmental responses. (In some groups, this can become a special problem in the observing wind-down at the end of session.) Emotional patterns they have not experienced, thought patterns they are not familiar with, and behaviors they have not exhibited are difficult for them to understand and validate. My experience, however, is that group members bend over backwards to validate one another and that a greater problem is for the leaders to draw out their negative observations and descriptions of one another. These negative reactions need also to be validated in the group setting. Peace at all costs, a typical objective in some borderline families, is not the norm in group skills training. Other clients, of course, grew up with the norm of no peace at any cost; once again, a dialectic emerges.

In group skills training sessions, validation means that the leaders should always point out the truth inherent in clients' comments and group experiences, even while simultaneously demonstrating the contradictory point of view. Conflict within the group or between an individual group member and a leader is dealt with by validating both sides of the conflict and arriving at a resolution that integrates both points of view, rather than invalidating one side or the other.

Change Procedures

Contingency Procedures

As noted in Chapter 3 of this manual, the major therapeutic contingencies are discussed in the first session when the rules of DBT skills training are introduced. However, only two of the rules involve clear contingencies: Missing 4 consecutive weeks of scheduled skills training sessions in a row, or not meeting with one's individual therapist for 4 consecutive weeks of scheduled sessions, will result in termination of therapy. There are no clear contingencies for violation of the other rules. In my experience, it is never a good idea to tell clients that they will be terminated from skills training if they break rules. So what are the contingencies for rule breaking? The main ones are therapist and/or member disapproval, attention to the rule breaking, more interpersonal distance and commitment from others, and loss of therapeutic effectiveness.

Contingency Management

As discussed in Chapter 10 of the text, the basic idea in contingency management is that the client's adaptive functional behavior should result in reinforcement and negative maladaptive behavior should result in either aversive outcomes or no discernible outcomes that could reinforce the behavior. The most important factors to keep in mind in applying contingencies are (1) that the outcomes for adaptive behaviors (i.e., all behaviors target for increase) must indeed be reinforcing for the particular client and (2) that principles of shaping must be taken into account. In skills training, therapists are faced with managing both in-session behaviors and behaviors that occur outside of sessions.

Applying reinforcing contingencies. The most important point to keep in mind here is that positive reinforcement must be impartially scrutinized. That is, skills trainers should not assume that a particular response on their part is a positive reinforcer without checking this out. One of the biggest mistakes therapists often make is to assume that public praise will reinforce client behaviors. In fact, public praise may serve to punish the very behaviors therapists are trying to increase. If an individual's history involves many instances in which praise and acknowledgment of skill and strength have led to an absence of further help, praise may come to alert the person to upcoming punishment or extinction. In my experience, this particular issue comes up over and over in skills training. It is not a good idea, however, to stop praising behaviors to be reinforced, because a client can interpret the absence of praise as her never being able to do anything right—in other words, as implied criticism. So what is the synthesis? The best strategy is to praise behavior appropriately (e.g., to comment that the behavior is skilled if it is, constitutes progress if it does, etc.) and to follow this immediately with a recognition that this does not mean that the client can solve all of her problems or has no more problems to be solved. In this way, the praise is freed from the expectancy that competence will result in loss of any further help. Use (and misuse) of praise as a reinforcer is discussed in more detail in Chapter 10 of the text.

As far as possible, skills trainers should try to provide natural reinforcers for clients' adaptive behavior. "Natural reinforcers" are responses that clients can expect in everyday life. Thus, if clients are taught assertion skills, and then trainers never reward assertive behaviors by giving them what they request, it is unreasonable to expect those behaviors to continue. Similarly, if clients' attempts at regulating intense emotions precipitated by having to talk in skills training sessions meet with the trainers' making them continue talking even longer, it is unreasonable to expect the clients to continue regulating their emotional responses. If clients improve their tolerance of aversive events during sessions, and this is followed by the trainers' reducing their efforts to make sessions less aversive, it is unreasonable to expect further distress tolerance. The point is that as clients begin to apply the skills being taught, skills trainers must be careful to respond in a manner that will reinforce such improvement. Although shaping principles require the trainers eventually to "up the ante," so to speak, and require even more skillful behavior, increases in demands must be kept gradual. Otherwise, clients will always feel that they cannot do enough to please the trainers or to get their needs met. It can also be useful to pair natural reinforcement with praise.

Extinction and Punishment Techniques. Even though reinforcement is the preferred form of contingency management, aversive (punishment) and extinction procedures are at times required. Generally, aversive procedures should be used when a client is trying to avoid difficult activities such as coming to skills training sessions, doing homework or in-session practice, or engaging in active problem solving. In these cases, it is essential to intervene immediately and push the client, instead of ignoring her and allowing the avoidance to continue. In other words, the avoidance response must be short-circuited. The idea is to make the immediate consequences of avoiding more aversive than those of not avoiding.

When a client misses a session, for example, the policy is to call her immediately and try to cheerlead her into coming to the session. The therapist uses the broken record strategy taught clients in the interpersonal skills module. (I usually have a bus schedule handy when I call.) The exception to this policy, discussed further on, is when calling reinforces missing sessions.

Another common avoidance pattern in a group context is for a member who did not do any homework practice to try not to discuss it in the session. If the group leaders jump over the member and go on to the next one, then the avoidance has worked. The best strategy is to move immediately, in a nonjudgmental and warm fashion, to an attempt to analyze not doing the homework. If the member still refuses after some pushing, the leader should move toward analyzing why she doesn't want to talk. The point is that avoidance should not be rewarded. When carried out fully, analysis of the resistance is an aversive technique for most clients.

Positive maladaptive behaviors (e.g., attempts to get attention, sobbing, hostile behavior, attempts to discuss weekly life crises) should be put on an extinction schedule. A skills trainer ignores the client's maladaptive behaviors and continues to interact with the client as if she is not producing such behaviors. Or, if the behaviors cannot be ignored, the trainer can make a brief comment suggesting that the client cope with her maladaptive behavior by using some of the skills she is learning in the current (or a past) skills module. Thus, a client who begins crying can be encouraged to practice her distress tolerance or mindfulness skills. If a client is storming out of the room, a trainer can suggest calmly that she attempt to use her emotion regulation skills and, once she is calm, come back into the session. Unless skills trainers have clear reasons to believe that a client is leaving a session to kill herself, clients should usually not be followed when they leave skills training sessions precipitously. (Even if it would not reinforce the person's leaving, it might serve as vicarious reinforcement for others' leaving.) However, leaving (and thus avoiding skills training) should not be reinforced unchecked. Thus, a trainer should alert the individual psychotherapist, so that the behavior can be dealt with in individual therapy as an instance of therapy-interfering behavior, or the precipitous leaving can be discussed in the next session.

It is very important to remember to soothe both clients whose behavior is on an extinction schedule and those who are receiving aversive consequences. (In my experience, the ability to put a client's behavior on an extinction schedule and simultaneously soothe the client is one of the hardest tasks to learn for new therapists.) In each case, the behavior is what is being punished, not the person. Especially in group skills training, leaders need to develop the ability to ignore many behaviors and to come back to the members with a soothing comment after the behaviors stop. Or, even while the dysfunctional behaviors are going on, leaders can soothe members while at the same time insisting that they practice their skills anyway. To a member crying about a relationship breakup, you might say something to this effect: "I know this is really difficult for you, but try your best to distract yourself from your troubles. Be mindful to the task and tell me about your efforts to practice your skills this week." After listening to a few other group members, the leader might go back to this member and ask briefly but warmly, "How are you doing with your attempt to be mindful to group? . . . Keep trying."

Shaping. Shaping is the backbone of skills training. Without shaping, both therapists and clients would become so frustrated and distressed that skills training could not proceed. Inevitably, borderline individuals have no self-shaping skills. Their unreasonable expectations for immediate perfection interfere constantly with their ability to learn the skills gradually. Thus, it is crucial that skills trainers continually model shaping principles. Not only should they be discussed openly and explained, but trainers' expectations of clients should also follow shaping principles. With the client in individual skills training, or the individual group member, the principles are no different than in individual therapy.

What group leaders sometimes forget, however, is that these same principles apply to the entire group. In my experience, one of the greatest difficulties in conducting DBT group skills training is that therapists' expectations for the group as a whole are far higher than the group can deliver. At our clinic it is not until the third year of therapy that borderline clients can interact in group sessions like reasonably ordinary group therapy clients.

Observing Limits

As I have discussed in Chapter 10 of the text, DBT does not generally believe in *setting* limits, but instead favors *observing* naturally occurring limits. In skills training, however, a number of limits are set by the therapy itself. These limits are arbitrary, in that I could conceivably have developed different rules. Other limits that must be observed are those of the skills trainers as individuals and (in a group context) of the group as a whole.

Limits of Skills Training. The key limitation of DBT skills training is that the skills trainers do not function as individual therapists during skills training sessions. The role of skills trainers is clearly defined and limited to teaching psychosocial skills and dealing with the interpersonal relationships that arise in sessions. A skills trainer is like a university professor or a high school teacher. "Personal" calls to skills training leaders are acceptable only under certain conditions. Clients may call if they will not be able to attend group for some reason, or if they have a serious interpersonal problem with a trainer that cannot be resolved in a session.

An exception to these phone limits occurs when a skills training client is also receiving DBT individual psychotherapy from another therapist in the same clinical setting. In these instances, a skills training leader serves as a backup therapist for the individual therapist. Thus, when the individual psychotherapist is out of town, it is appropriate for the client to call the skills training therapist under the same circumstances that she would call her individual therapist. When the reason for the call is to discuss interpersonal relationships in the skills training, there are some limits. These limits are the natural limits of the skills training leader, and thus the ordinary strategies of observing limits in individual therapy apply. It is essential that a skills training leader in this situation understand these phone limits and communicate them clearly to the clients.

In my experience, the best way to communicate phone limits is by discussing the important role of the individual psychotherapist in the total DBT program, and pointing out that skills trainers do not duplicate the individual psychotherapist's job. In our experience, clients grasp this rule very quickly and rarely violate it. Most phone calls other than session cancellations revolve around their relationships with skills trainers or (in a group context) with other group members. At times a client may call to find out whether a trainer hates her and wants her out of skills training. At other times a client may call to discuss how it is completely impossible to continue in skills training any longer, since sessions are so painful. Relationship problem-solving strategies must be implemented by the skills training leaders during such phone calls. These are discussed in detail both in Chapter 15 of the text and at the end of this chapter.

A second limit during the first year of DBT skills training is that personal crises are generally not discussed in skills training sessions. This limit is made crystal clear for the first several sessions and is reclarified thereafter when clients wish to discuss their current crises. If a crisis is extreme, of course, skills training leaders may choose to violate the rule. To cite a very extreme example, when a group member in our clinic was raped on her way to a group session, we of course discussed it. A death in the family, a divorce, a breakup of a relationship, or a rejection by a therapist may be reported and briefly discussed at the beginning of sessions.

The key to getting borderline individuals to follow this rule is in how a crisis is dealt with. Generally, any topic can be discussed if the focus is on how the client can use the skills being learned to cope with the crisis. Thus, although at first glance it would appear that the "crisis of the week" cannot be discussed, at second glance it is obvious that it can be, as long as it is discussed within the context of DBT skills. This orientation, however, is not always the orientation that a person is hoping for. Rather than giving clients free rein to discuss their problems and to share all the details, skills training leaders very quickly intervene to highlight the relationship of these problems to the particular skill module of the moment.

For example, if an individual psychotherapist has terminated a client, this can be dealt with in terms of the interpersonal effectiveness skills the client can use to find out why, to find a new therapist, or to get her therapist back. It can also be approached from the standpoint of how hurt the client is feeling in response to the rejection and how the client can feel better. If core mindfulness skills are the focus, the client can be encouraged to observe and describe the event and her responses. She can also be helped to notice whether she is judging and how she can focus on what works rather than on revenge. Finally, the problem can be approached in terms of how the person is going to survive it or tolerate it without engaging in impulsive destructive behaviors. Most problems lend themselves to an analysis in terms of each of the skill modules. Noninterpersonal situations which at first glance may seem inappropriate for the interpersonal effectiveness module, can be looked at as opportunities for finding friends to share with and for obtaining the social support the client needs to cope with the problem. Skills trainers must be vigilant in always bringing the crisis back to the skills. When the skills seem ineffective or insufficient for the problem, the client should be encouraged to talk with her individual therapist.

Finally, the limits of structured skills training may have to be observed in regard to process issues. Some clients in a group context are more than happy to have group sessions run in a psychoeducational format rather than an interpersonal process format. However, in every group I have ever run, a number of people are very dissatisfied with this approach and are far more comfortable discussing interpersonal problems and group issues. Such patients will inevitably suggest that skills training is not "real therapy" if these problems are not addressed. The group leaders need to carefully communicate the limits of skills training versus psychotherapy on this point. (The tendency to favor process discussions and work on individual crises is, as I have noted previously, much more pronounced when skills training is conducted individually and is a principal reason for conducting skills training in groups.)

Personal Limits of Skills Training Leaders. The observing-limits approach with respect to the skills training leaders is no different in DBT skills training than it is in other components of DBT. Essentially, it is the task of the leaders to observe their own limits in conducting the treatment. In my experience, the crucial limit that must be observed has to do with phone calls. Therapists must track their own ability to handle lengthy interpersonal discussions with clients and must communicate their limits clearly to the clients.

Limits of a Group as a Whole. The key limit of first-year DBT skills training groups is that they cannot tolerate hostile attacks in sessions. My colleagues and I have had to make it very clear with group members that such behaviors as throwing things, destroying property, and attacking or harshly criticizing other group members are proscribed. When hostile behavior occurs, group members are encouraged to work on the problem with their individual psychotherapists. However, it is preferable for an individual to leave a group session (even if only temporarily) than to engage in these behaviors. The group leaders, of course have to be careful in this situation not to punish the member for leaving on the one hand and to punish her for staying on the other. Dialectical balance is crucial, since the leaders also want to encourage the member to stay at a session and inhibit maladaptive behaviors as long as possible.

Exposure-Based Procedures

Structured exposure-based procedures are not used in DBT skills training, although there is no reason why ancillary treatments oriented to exposure (e.g., sexual abuse groups) could not be combined effectively with DBT. Less structured exposure-based procedures, however, are consistently used in skills training in two ways. First, clients' avoidance of topics, procedures, and process discussions (when process is the focus) is almost always blocked. Second, clients are instructed over and over about the value of exposure. In well-run DBT skills training, after several months of therapy every client should be able to give a very good rationale for why and when avoidance makes things worse and why and when exposure improves them. Thus, when clients employ exposure to difficult tasks or feared situations during homework practice, the therapists should note and reinforce it.

Cognitive Modification Procedures

Cognitive Restructuring

There are a number of structured exercises throughout the skills training program for helping clients examine and modify dysfunctional assumptions and beliefs. However, formal cognitive restructuring plays a much smaller role in DBT than in other forms of cognitive–behavioral treatments, and cognitive treatment of BPD in particular. This topic is discussed extensively in Chapters 8 and 11 of the text.

Contingency Clarification

The task in contingency clarification is to help patients clarify the "if–then" contingency relationships in their lives and in the therapy situation. Contingency clarification can be distinguished from the didactic strategies. The didactic strategies stress general contingent rules that hold for all or most people, contingency clarification always looks for the contingent relationships operating in an individual client's life.

One of the reasons for the moment-to-moment, point-to-point exploration during behavioral analysis is to help clients learn to better observe the contingent relationships occurring in their everyday lives. Borderline individuals often have great difficulty observing these natural contingencies. When it comes to observing the effects of using new behavioral skills, they may be motivated to miss the benefits. The dialectic here is between being competent and getting help — a point discussed in the preceding chapter. One of the skills trainers' tasks here is to demonstrate to clients that the contingencies formerly favoring dysfunctional behaviors are not currently operating. Thus, whereas it may have previously been true that when a client acted in a capable manner she lost her access to help, the rule is no longer operat-

ing in skills training. I discuss the clarification of therapeutic contingencies further at the end of this chapter.

In the interpersonal effectiveness module, it is important to stress the importance of observing contingencies in interpersonal encounters. Thus, homework practice always includes trying a new skill and observing its outcome. The idea is not to prove preconceived beliefs of the therapists or the clients about contingent relationships, but rather to explore the actual contingent relationships naturally existing in the client's everyday lives. It will often become clear in the process that contingencies or rules for one person may not apply to another. Furthermore, rules that operate in one context may not operate in another for the very same person.

Figuring out the rules of the game, so to speak, is intimately related to the behavioral skill of being effective or focusing on what works—one of the core mindfulness skills. Focusing on what works is focusing on engaging in behaviors where contingent outcomes are the desired outcomes. This approach is often a new one for borderline individuals, since they are more experienced at looking at behaviors in terms of "right" or "wrong" from a moral point of view than in terms of outcomes or consequences. Contingency clarification strategies are a step in moving these individuals toward more effective behavior.

In discussing behavioral outcomes, skills trainers should remember that a poor outcome is not necessarily proof that a particular skill does not work, and should examine carefully whether the person actually performed the skilled behavior correctly. At times, a person will say that a particular response does not help when the problem is that the individual could not produce the skilled response. This is a very tricky distinction and requires patience and care during behavioral analysis.

Stylistic Strategies

Reciprocal Communication Strategies

Reciprocal communication in the context of skills training requires that trainers make themselves vulnerable to their clients and express this vulnerability in a manner that can be heard and understood by the clients. As always, there is a question of balance here, and the fulcrum on which this balance is based is the therapeutic welfare of the clients. Thus, reciprocity is in the service of the clients, not for the benefit of the skills training leaders. Leaders' expression of vulnerability in sessions not only addresses the power imbalance that all clients experience, but also can serve as an important modeling event: It can teach clients how to draw the line between privacy and sharing, how to experience vulnerable states without shame, and how to cope with their own limitations. In addition, it provides a glimpse into the world of so-called "normal" people, thus normalizing vulnerability and life with limitations.

One of the easiest ways to use reciprocal communication in skills training is for the skills trainers to share their own experiences in doing homework practice. In my experience, one of the benefits of leading skill groups is that it gives me an opportunity to also work on improving my own skills. If group leaders can share their own attempts (and especially their failures) with humor, so much the better. Sometimes, the trick is for the leaders to label their own experiences as relevant to the skills the group is attempting to learn. For example, when I am teaching how to say no to unwanted requests, I almost always discuss my own difficulties in saying no to group members' pressures to get me to do things I don't think are therapeutic. Since resisting their intense attempts at persuasion usually requires me to use all of my own skills, the example covers quite a bit of the material we teach in skills training. By now, all of my skills groups know about my efforts to deal with my unreasonable fear of heights when I go hiking (focusing on one thing in the moment, distraction, self-encouragement), with back pain on meditation retreats (focusing on one thing, radical acceptance), and with other assorted life dilemmas I encounter from week to week. Coleaders of mine have discussed their troubles in learning to meditate, difficulties with asking for things, problems in coping with bosses and professors, the process of mourning losses, and so on. The point is that sharing one's own flawed attempts to use the skills being taught can provide valuable modeling both in how to apply skills and in how to respond to one's own vulnerability in a nonjudgmental fashion.

Reciprocal communication can be especially difficult to practice in a group setting as opposed to a one-to-one setting. It can feel like many against one or two. This difficulty, of course, should give group leaders more empathy for the group members, who usually experience the very same problem. Nonetheless, sharing the difficulty does not make it go away. It can also be very difficult to respond in a manner appropriate to each member, when members are in many different places (psychologically speaking) at once. The time it takes to find out where even one member is may preclude efforts to explore the current psychological state of other members. And, to the extent that group leaders attend to such within-session process issues, they are veering away from the goals of skills training anyway. By contrast, as an individual therapist you can titrate responses to fit the individual client; timing and attention to various topics can be geared to the state of the one person at hand.

In group sessions, it is very difficult to strike a response that meets each member's needs. Thus, it is often much more difficult to move the group forward (or anywhere but down, it often seems). This frustration may act to make group leaders want to pull away and close up, or, at other times, to pull close enough to attack. Either way, the frustration reduces the experience of warmth and engagement. In such a stressful atmosphere, it is sometimes difficult to relax. And it is difficult for leaders to be responsive when they are not relaxed.

Great care must be taken to observe the effects of self-disclosure on group members. To a certain extent, their ability to accept such a stance is variable. In a group setting, however, individual differences may be harder to detect than in the individual setting, where the focus is always on the individual client. Difficulties are easy to camouflage and easy to overlook. It can be reasonably safely said, however, that all members will have difficulties with the leaders' expressing their frustration and/or anger with the group; thus, extraordinary care must be taken in doing so.

Irreverent Communication Strategies

Irreverence has to be used very carefully in group skills training, although it can be used quite liberally when skills training is conducted individually. This is because irreverence requires a therapist to observe very closely the immediate effects of his or her response and move to repair any damage as quickly as possible. It is very difficult to be that astute and attentive to each individual in a group setting. The person a group leader is talking to may be very receptive to an irreverent statement, but another group member, listening in, may be horrified. Once leaders get to know their clients fairly well, they can be more comfortable using irreverence. Specific examples and the rationale for the irreverent communication are discussed in Chapter 12 of the text.

The main place for irreverence, in a group context, is usually in the individual work with each client during the first hour of a session (the practice-sharing component). In irreverence, problematic behavior is reacted to as if it were normal, and functional adaptive behavior is reacted to with enthusiasm, vigor, and positive emotionality. Or dysfunctional plans or actions may be overreacted to in a humorous fashion. Or behaviors or communications may be responded to in a blunt, confrontational style. The aim of irreverence is to jolt the individual client, or the group as a whole, into seeing things from a new, more enlightened perspective. Irreverent communication should help clients to make the transition from seeing their own dysfunctional behavior as a cause of shame and scorn to seeing it as inconsequential and even funny and humorous. To do this, a therapist can only be a half step ahead of them; timing is of the essence. An irreverent attitude is not an insensitive attitude, nor is it an excuse for hostile or demeaning behavior. A group leader always takes suffering seriously, albeit matter-of-factly, calmly, and sometimes with humor.

Case Management Strategies

Environmental Intervention Strategies

Environmental intervention strategies are almost never used by the therapists in skills training. Members of a skills training group, however, are encouraged to use these strategies with one another. For example, clients are encouraged to call one another when in trouble, ask favors of one another, get rides to group meetings or to hospitals when needed, and so forth. Clients will often want much more environmental intervention from skills trainers than the trainers should be willing to give. An example (which occurs frequently) has to do with getting a pass from an inpatient unit to come to a session. It can often be difficult for a client to talk a hospital into giving such a pass. The client may then want a skills trainer to call the hospital on her behalf.

The trainer's first response should be to emphasize to the client that it is her responsibility to behave in such a way that inpatient treatment personnel will want to let her leave the hospital on a pass for skills training. My one concession to the politics of inpatient hospitalization is that if it appears absolutely necessary, I will call the inpatient personnel to let them know that I do indeed expect that inpatients get themselves out on a pass to come to skills training sessions. I do not, however, try to convince them to let a particular client out. Over and over in skills training, sessions trainers must stress that their job is to teach clients environmental intervention skills so that they can do environmental interventions for themselves. New clients may be shocked at first with this confidence that they will eventually succeed in learning these skills. But the shock is balanced with an emerging pleasure at being treated as adults who can run their own lives.

Consultation-to-the-Patient/ Client Strategies

In general, DBT requires a skills training therapist to play the role of a consultant to the client rather than that of a consultant to other people in the client's social network, including other therapists the client may have. DBT assumes that the client is capable of performing intermediary functions between various therapists. Thus, the skills training therapist does not play a parental role, assuming that the client is unable to communicate in a straightforward manner with those in her own treatment network. When safety is an immediate issue, or it is very obvious that the client cannot serve as an intermediary for herself, the therapist should move from the "consultation-to-the-patient" (or, in this context, "client") strategies to the environmental intervention strategies. Rules for when to use which of the two group of strategies are clearly laid out in Chapter 13 of the text. The consultation strategies are quite different from how therapists may have learned to relate to other professionals treating their clients. The rationale for the strategies is spelled out in the text as well.

The one exception to these rules occurs when an individual in skills training is in a complete DBT program, including DBT individual psychotherapy. In such a case, the client's skills training and individual therapists consult weekly. The role of the skills trainers in these consultations is to give the individual psychotherapist information about how the client is doing in skills training; they alert him or her to problems that may need work in individual psychotherapy and share insights that are being given in the skills training sessions.

These consultations are limited to sharing of information and joint treatment planning. It must, of course, be clear to the client from the very beginning that she is being treated by a team of therapists who will coordinate therapy at every opportunity. The interaction of the two therapy modalities is stressed by both the individual and the skills training therapists. A DBT skills training therapist, however, does not serve as an intermediary for the individual client with her individual psychotherapist. If she is having problems with her individual therapist, the skills training leaders should usually consult with her on how she might address these problems in the individual therapy. Generally, the task of the skills training therapists here is to help the client use the skills she is learning to work on the problem.

If a client is in individual therapy that is independent of the DBT skills training program (i.e., with another therapist in a different treatment setting), the consultation-to-the-client approach will generally involve some contact with the individual therapist. These consultations ordinarily should not be conducted without the client present. The material taught in skills training can and usually should be shared with the individual psychotherapist. The skills trainers' task in this case is to help the client do this effectively.

Difficulties that individual clients experience with other therapists and clinical agencies can be dealt with in the skills training sessions if those difficulties can be made relevant to the skills being taught. Thus, in the interpersonal effectiveness module, an individual client may be helped to communicate more effectively with other professionals treating her. In the emotion regulation module, she can be helped to modulate her emotional reactions to these professionals. During the distress tolerance module, she can be assisted in accepting and tolerating the behaviors of other professionals that she finds problematic. Generally, problems with treatment professionals brought up in skills training sessions are dealt with in precisely the same manner that any other interpersonal problem is dealt with.

Special Treatment Strategies

There are six integrative strategies in DBT for responding to the following specific issues and problems in treatment: crises, suicidal behavior, therapy-interfering behavior, telephone calls, ancillary treatments, and therapeutic relationship issues. I have discussed the telephone strategies for skills trainers earlier in this chapter. And in a standard DBT program, teaching clients to utilize ancillary treatments (medication, inpatient hospitalization, etc.) effectively is the responsibility of their individual therapists and not the skills trainers (see Chapter 15 of the text for a discussion).

In the remainder of this chapter, I review the crisis, suicidal behavior, and therapy-interfering behavior strategies as they apply to skills training. I have covered these three sets of strategies in such detail in the text, however, that I discuss them briefly here. The relationship strategies, on the other hand, require a good deal more work in a group skills training context; thus, I discuss them at some length.

Crisis Strategies

The responsibility for assisting a client in crisis belongs to the primary or individual psychotherapist. When a skills training client is in crisis, a skills trainer should (1) refer her to her psychotherapist, assisting her in making contact if necessary, and (2) help her apply distress tolerance skills until she makes contact. The crisis strategies described in Chapter 15 of the text should be used in a modified version.

Just as borderline clients are often in a state of individual crisis, a group can be in a state of crisis also. A group in crisis is functioning in a state of emotional overload. Usually, this will be the result of a common trauma such as a group member's committing suicide, a hostile act directed at the entire group, a therapist's leaving, and so on. In these instances, group leaders should employ all of the crisis strategies used in individual crisis intervention; they are simply applied to the entire group instead of to one client. The steps are summarized in Table 5.1.

TABLE 5.1. Crisis Strategies Checklist (Group Context)

____ T attends to emotion rather than content.
____ T explores the problem now.
    ____ T focuses on immediate time frame.
    ____ T identifies key events setting off current emotions and sense of crisis.
    ____ T formulates and summarizes the problem.
____ T focuses on problem solving.
____ T gives advice and makes suggestions.
____ T frames possible solutions in terms the skills group is learning.
    ____ T predicts future consequences of action plans.
    ____ T confronts group maladaptive ideas or behavior directly.
    ____ T clarifies and reinforces group's adaptive responses.
    ____ T identifies factors interfering with productive plans of action.
____ T focuses on affect tolerance.
____ T helps group commit itself to a plan of action.
____ T assesses group members' suicide risk (if necessary).
____ T anticipates a recurrence of the crisis response.

Note. In this table and Tables 5.2 and 5.3, T refers to the skills training therapist.

Suicidal Behavior Strategies

If the risk of suicide is imminent (Tables 15.3 and 15.4 in Chapter 15 of the text provide the information needed to assess this), a skills trainer should call the individual psychotherapist immediately for instructions on how to proceed. During periods of crises and high suicide risk, it may be useful to ask the individual therapist to be on call following group sessions. If the individual therapist cannot be located, the skills trainer must do crisis intervention until contact can be made with the individual therapist. Generally, a skills trainer should be much more conservative in the treatment of suicidal risk than is the individual therapist. It is essential, however, to get and keep a copy of the individual therapist's crisis planning sheet (see Figure 15.1 in the text).

Steps for intervention when a client is threatening imminent suicide or parasuicide, or is actually engaging in parasuicidal behavior during contact (or has just engaged in it), are listed in Table 5.2. They are discussed in detail in the text.

Therapy-Destructive and Therapy-Interfering Behavior Strategies

When a client is engaging in behaviors that are clearly destructive to skills training, the skills trainers must respond promptly and vigorously. A modified version of the therapy-interfering behavior protocol described in Chapter 15 of the text can be applied here; the strategies, modified for use in a skills training setting, are listed in Table 5.3.

TABLE 5.2. Suicidal Behavior Strategies Checklist

When threats of imminent suicide or parasuicide are occurring and T cannot turn management over to individual psychotherapist

_____ T assesses the risk of suicide and of parasuicide.

_____ T uses known factors related to imminent suicidal behavior to predict imminent risk.

_____ T uses a crisis planning sheet.

_____ T knows the likely lethality of various suicide/parasuicide methods.

_____ T consults with emergency services or medical consultant about medical risk of planned and/or available method(s). T is more conservative than in individual psychotherapy.

_____ T removes or gets C to remove lethal items.

_____ T emphatically instructs C not to commit suicide or engage in parasuicide.

_____ T maintains a position that suicide is not a good solution.

_____ T generates hopeful statements and solutions for coping until contact with individual therapist can be made.

_____ T keeps contact when suicide risk is imminent and high, until C's care can be transferred to individual therapist.

_____ T anticipates a recurrence before contact is made with individual therapist.

_____ T communicates C's suicide risk to individual therapist as soon as possible.

When a parasuicidal act is taking place during contact or has just taken place.

_____ T assesses potential medical risk of behavior, consulting with local emergency services or other medical resources to determine risk when necessary.

_____ T assesses C's ability to obtain medical treatment on her own.

_____ If medical emergency exists, T alerts individuals near C and calls emergency services.

_____ T stays in contact with C until aid arrives.

_____ T calls individual therapist.

_____ If risk is low, T instructs C to obtain medical treatment, if necessary, and to call her individual therapist.

Note. In this table and Table 5.3, C refers to the client.

TABLE 5.3. Therapy-Destructive Behavior Strategies Checklist

_____ T behaviorally defines what C is doing to destroy therapy.

_____ T conducts a brief analysis of destructive behavior.

_____ T refers C to her individual psychotherapist for an in-depth behavioral analysis of the destructive behavior.

_____ T makes contingencies very clear for continued destructive behaviors.

_____ T adopts a problem-solving plan with C.

_____ When C refuses to modify behavior:

_____ T discusses goals of therapy with C.

_____ T avoids unnecessary power struggles.

_____ T considers a vacation from therapy until behavior comes under control.

When a therapy-interfering behavior is failure to do homework practice assignments, it is responded to during homework practice review. I have already discussed this in previous sections of this chapter. With most other therapy interfering behaviors, skills trainers should use the therapy-destructive behavior strategies in Table 5.3 in a more gentle manner, or the relationship problem-solving strategies discussed below.

Relationship Strategies

Relationship Acceptance

Relationship acceptance in group skills training requires that leaders experience and communicate acceptance of group members in several different spheres. First, as in individual therapy, the clinical progress of each client must be accepted as it is. Relationships between leaders and group members, between members and other therapists, between and among individual members, between the group leaders themselves, and between the group as a whole and the group leaders must also be accepted. The sheer complexity of the situation can make acceptance difficult, because it is easy to get overwhelmed; rigidity and nonacceptance usually follow. It is essential to try not to pave over or quickly truncate conflict and difficult emotions in the group. Many borderline clients have great difficulty with group skills training. Some are in it only because it is required, and they feel uncomfortable and are unable to interact effectively in this atmosphere. For others, skills seem unimportant, juvenile, or silly. Still others quickly become demoralized by unsuccessful attempts to master the skills.

Group skills training with borderline clients does not have the naturally occurring characteristics reinforcing leaders that most groups have. Skills training leaders are faced with dead silences; noncompliance; inappropriate and sometimes extreme responses to the slightest deviation from perfect sensitivity; and a group atmosphere that at times can be noncommunicative, hostile, nonsupportive, and nonappreciative. The potential for mistakes in leading such a group is vast. A leader can expect not only to make many, but to be acutely aware of many of the mistakes the other group leader makes. Reality acceptance skills are crucial if mistakes are to be responded to in a nondestructive manner.

Attacking group members, or threatening them, is almost always a result of a failure of relationship acceptance. Acceptance requires a nonjudgmental attitude that sees all problems as part of the therapeutic process—"grist for the mill," so to speak. Leaders simply have to see that most problematic responses on the part of the group are derivative responses based on borderline response patterns. In other words, if borderline clients didn't present with the problems that drive leaders crazy, they wouldn't need a skills training group. To the extent that leaders fail to recognize this fact, they are likely to engage in rejecting, victim-bashing behaviors that may be too subtle to be seen for what they are, but nonetheless have an iatrogenic effect. In other words, an "easy" leader disposition has to either be innate or cultivated.

Relationship Enhancement

Relationship enhancement strategies (discussed briefly in connection with contracting strategies in Chapter 14 of the text) have to do with a therapist's behaviors that increase therapeutic values of the relationship. These are those behaviors that make the relationship more than simply a helpful friendship. A positive collaborative interpersonal relationship is no less important in skills training than it is in individual psychotherapy. However, the development of such a relationship is considerably more complex in group skills training because of the increased number of individuals involved in the relationship. The question for the group leaders is how to establish such a relationship both between group members and leaders and among the members themselves.

All of the DBT strategies are designed in one way or another to enhance the collaborative working relationship. The strategies discussed here are those intended primarily to establish the group leaders as experts, as creditable, and as efficacious. Thus, the goal of these strategies is to communicate to the group members that the leaders indeed know what they are doing and have something to offer that will probably be helpful to the group members. This is no easy task. The task is made even more difficult by the fact that group members often share with one another their previous failures in both individual and other group therapies, and comment about the hopelessness of their situation and the meagerness of any help that can be offered. Group members often portray their problems as Goliath and the treatment as David, but without David ending as he does in the Old Testament. The task of the leaders is to convey the story as it indeed occurred.

Expertise, credibility, and efficacy can be conveyed in a variety of ways. Therapists' neatness, professionalism, interest, comfort, self-confidence, speech style, and preparation for therapy sessions are no less useful in skills training than in individual psychotherapy. It is especially important in conducting groups to have the group room prepared before the group members arrive: Forms should be distributed, chairs should be in place, and the refreshments should be made. The key to the credibility problem, in my experience, is that clients simply do not believe that learning the skills presented will in fact be helpful. This disbelief detracts from any positive motivation to learn the skills, and unless clients learn the skills and obtain positive rewards it is difficult to change this attitude. Thus, it is a vicious circle.

Leaders must come up with a way to break this vicious circle if the clients are to move. The most helpful approach is simply for the leaders to tell group members that in their experience these skills have been helpful to some people some of the time. This, of course, can only be said if that is indeed the leaders' experience; leaders who have never taught these skills must rely on others' experience. (Our outcome data can form a data base for inexperienced therapists.) In addition, leaders can share their own experience with skills. For some clients, the most powerful inducement to learn the skills is the knowledge that the leaders have found the skills helpful for themselves.

Credibility is damaged when leaders promise that a particular skill will solve a particular problem. In fact, DBT is something of a shotgun approach: Some of the skills work some of the time for some of the people. I have not had any clients to date who could not benefit from something, but no one benefits from everything. It is crucial to present this information; otherwise the leaders' credibility is on the line immediately.

Another key issue to address is that of trust and confidentiality. Opportunities to display trustworthiness occur when one member is absent from a group session. At all times, confidences must be kept and unnecessary information about a group member should not be conveyed when that group member is absent. The absence of a group member, however, can serve as a powerful opportunity for enhancing other group members' trust in the leaders. The manner in which the absent member is discussed conveys information to all other members about how they will be treated when they are absent. Generally, the policy should be to protect group members from negative judgments. For example, if a group member blows up and walks out of a session, the leaders can respond to the event with sympathetic explanations of her behavior rather than with critical judgments of her walking out.

This same strategy, of course, can be used when all group members are present. It is not unusual for one group member to behave in a fashion that the leaders know will result in negative judgments by other group members. Or other group members may be quite critical of one another. The leaders' role here is that of protectors of the accused and the judged. This leader task cannot be over stressed, especially during the client's first year of skills training. Not only does this approach serve to model nonjudgmental observation and description of problematic behavior for group members, but it also conveys to all of the members that when attacked they too will be protected.

The most useful way to convey expertness and credibility is, of course, to be helpful. Thus, the leaders need to think through skills that have a high likelihood of working with a particular group member. A skill that is working should be highlighted so that the member will also see the benefits.

Therapist credibility in standard DBT group skills training is further complicated by the fact that there are two group leaders. In my clinic, the coleader is usually a trainee who, in fact, does not have the expertise of the primary leader. It is essential that the primary leader not undermine the credibility and expertness of the coleader. It is important for the inexperienced coleader to find his or her emotional center and act from there. It is this innercenteredness, rather than any particular set of therapeutic skills, that is most important. The primary leader and coleader do not need to have the same set of skills or to convey expertise in the same areas. The dialectical perspective on the whole is what counts.

Relationship Problem Solving

Relationship problem solving is the application of general problem-solving strategies to the therapeutic relationship. In individual skills training, that relationship is between the trainer and the client. In group skills training, however, at least four relationships may require problem solving: member versus group leader, group versus group leader, member versus member, and leader versus leader. Not only are there more relationships to balance, but there are also many more issues coming into play. The public nature of the relationships is particularly important. Borderline individuals are exquisitely sensitive to any threat of rejection or criticism; when that rejection or criticism is public, they may experience such overwhelming and intense shame that it completely cuts off any chance of adequate problem solving. Thus, leaders have to be correspondingly sensitive in dealing with relationship problems in first-year DBT skills training groups. The relationship problem solving typical of process therapy groups is simply not possible in the beginning. Therefore, some of this problem solving has to be conducted individually and outside of the group sessions. Otherwise, problems may not be resolved and may escalate to such an extent that members find it impossible to continue in the group.

Member versus Group Leader. It is essential for a borderline client to form an attached relationship with at least one of the group leaders if she is to continue in skills training. Without such an attachment, the trials, tribulations, and traumas that frequently arise in skills training will simply overwhelm the client, and she will eventually drop out of therapy. This individual relationship, which is distinct from a leader's relationship to the group as a whole, is enhanced by individual attention given to group members before and after group meetings and during breaks.

When interpersonal problems with a group leader arise during the first year, they almost always must be solved outside of group meetings. Depending on the seriousness of the problem, a problem-solving meeting may take place on the phone or in a scheduled individual session before or after a group meeting. Whenever possible, such an individual meeting should be scheduled near in time to the group session, so that it does not take on the character of an individual psychotherapy. It is best to hold the meeting in a corner of the group therapy room. Also, the focus should be kept on the member's problems with the group or with the leader. In these individual meetings, the same relationship problem-solving strategies are utilized as in individual psychotherapy.

As a first step, the leader should help the group member observe and describe exactly what the problem is and with whom she has the problem. Sometimes, the problem will be with one or the other of the leaders. The public light of group sessions seems to enhance member sensitivity to even slight rejections or insensitive comments on the part of the leaders. Comments that might not lead to trouble in individual psychotherapy can lead to great problems in group therapy. Thus, if the problem is a leader's behavior, problem solving should be centered around it.

At other times, however, the problem is not with a group leader's behavior, but rather with the notion of attending and working in the group at all. Although these problems usually are dealt with in DBT individual psychotherapy (it must be kept in mind that the primary therapist assists the client with all behaviors that interfere with treatment, including those that show up in ancillary or collateral treatment), at times a client may profit from some individual attention from the group leaders also. During these meetings, strategies can be worked out to reduce the stress on the individual member. For example, we have had some group members who simply could not sit through an entire group session without becoming hostile or having a panic attack. In these cases, plans were developed so that when the clients saw that their behavior was about to go out of control, they would get up and leave the session for a few moments' break. Such a plan could have been worked out by clients' individual psychotherapists as well.

Careful attention must be paid to issues of shaping. Borderline clients are prone to indirect communication which at times requires mindreading on their therapists' part. How much mindreading should a group skills training therapist engage in, and how much reaching out to a withdrawn group member should occur?

As with individual psychotherapy, the goal is to require the group member to reach up to her capability and if possible slightly beyond, without requiring so much that she falls back in failure. At the beginning of the year, leaders will often need to telephone group members when they miss sessions or after they storm out of sessions.

The key, however, is not to engage in this behavior so reliably that the client begins to expect it, count on it, and become distressed if a leader does not reach out or call. The best approach here is for leaders to be direct in their communications about what they will and won't do. As discussed earlier in this Chapter, the DBT policy is to reach out and call group members when such calling is not reinforcing maladaptive behaviors, and to refrain from reaching out when it will reinforce such behaviors. Obviously, such judgments are difficult. It is especially difficult at the beginning of skills training, when leaders have little idea of the group members' respective capabilities; in this case, it is important to make policies clear. In all cases, however, it is essential not to *assume* that a particular response on the part of the leaders is reinforcing. There is no substitute for observing the consequences of various therapeutic actions.

Generally, our policies are as follows. If a member does not show up for a skills training session the person is called immediately by one of the leaders and urged strongly to drop everything and come to the group session immediately. This phone call is designed to cut off the person's ability to avoid a group session. The average borderline client believes that if she doesn't come to a group session, she won't have to deal with group issues; calling her immediately interferes with the avoidance. The phone conversation should be strictly kept to a discussion of how the person can get herself to the session, even if she arrives for only the last half hour. We have at times even offered to send a leader out to pick a person up when her reason for not coming is lack of transportation. In short, the phone call in this situation serves to cut off reinforcement for avoidance rather than to reinforce the avoidance behavior.

If a leader waits a few days to call, however, or if the phone call addresses the person's problems, then the call may well reinforce the client's tendency to withdraw rather than confront problems. In this event, the withdrawal leads to positive outreach on the part of the therapist, a positive interaction and sometimes a positive resolution. The dialectical dilemma here is the need to choose between avoiding reinforcing withdrawal and allowing a member to drop out. A leader simply has to face the fact that many borderline clients cannot engage in problem solving alone. Thus, in the interests of shaping, the leader should call and do problem solving and should then highlight that the direct discussion of the problem does result in problem resolution. Once this pattern is stabilized, then the leader can gradually decrease the degree of outreach while simultaneously verbally instructing the individual that she is expected to increase her outreach to the leaders and to the skills training group. Thus, while at the beginning the leader walks all the way over to the client's side of the teeter-totter, he or she needs to grab the client and begin moving back toward the middle. Without this movement, the very problems that outreach is intended to resolve may be exacerbated.

During the first 6 months, leaders should expect to spend a considerable amount of time resolving crises related to skills training. The key point, though, is that interventions should be limited to the clients' relationship to the group as a whole or to the group leaders. In other crisis situations, leaders should instruct the clients to call their individual therapists. If a leader suspects that phone calls may be reinforcing a client's problem, outcomes of phone calls should be closely observed, and the possibility should be discussed openly with the client as yet another problem to be solved.

Because there are two leaders in group skills training, each leader should take great care to observe the consultation-to-the-client approach. That is, one leader should not become an intermediary between a client and the other leader. A leader can, however, work with the client about how to resolve a problem with the other leader. In my experience, it is rare for a group member to be having serious problems with both group leaders at the same time. When this occurs, the DBT individual therapist must be a consultant to the client.

The most important idea here is that relationship problems between group members and group leaders should not be ignored. When these problems are serious or long-standing, they usually cannot be resolved during group skills training sessions. In fact, a major difference between our second- and third-year process groups and our first-year skills training groups is this very point. The goal of second- and third-year process groups is for clients to begin developing the ability to engage in relationship problem solving during group sessions. Thus, skills training leaders should expect to spend a considerable amount of time during the first several months of therapy interacting individually with group members before and after sessions and during breaks. In my experience, if a balance can be struck between reaching out when needed and drawing a member in simultaneously, most problems can be resolved. Ignoring the problems almost never makes them go away.

The most difficult problem to address and the easiest to ignore is that of the group member who comes to every session and stays for the entire session, but either interacts in a hostile manner or withdraws. Once I had a group member who came and fell asleep during most group sessions. What I wanted to do was reciprocally withdraw from the group member. When a leader withdraws from a group member, however, the group member can be expected to withdraw even further and eventually drop out. Addressing these issues directly in group sessions can be so threatening that it is almost never a good idea in the first year, at least not as a first approach. Since the group member is not directly expressing a problem and is not asking for attention, it is the leader's responsibility to approach her and set up an individual consultation before or after a group session or during the break.

Failure to initiate an action is usually a sign that a leader is frustrated and is, perhaps not motivated to keep the member in the group. At these times, having a second leader can be an enormous asset. The one leader can prod the other to address the issue.

Group versus Group Leaders. When the entire group is engaging in therapy-interfering behavior vis-à-vis the group leaders, the problem cannot, of course, be dealt with individually; it is a group problem. When should this problem be addressed directly, and when should it be ignored? An attempt to address the problem directly often backfires. Once group members have withdrawn or begun to interact in a hostile manner, they are often unable to stop the withdrawal in order to process the problem. Any move on the leaders' part to address the problem is viewed as criticizing further or as creating more conflict, and the group simply withdraws further.

It is usually better either to ignore the group withdrawal or hostility, or to comment on it briefly without pushing the issue and then focus on drawing out individual group members. At this point, it is essential to be able to cajole, distract, and otherwise respond to the problem in a relatively indirect manner. If leaders reciprocate with hostility, coldness, and withdrawal the problem will increase.

This is perhaps one of the most difficult situations that group skills training leaders must face. Unfortunately, it is also a very common situation in the beginning months of group skills training. It is a bit like trying to walk through quicksand—pulling with all one's strength to get one foot up, and then putting it down again in front of the other. Although it is exhausting and frustrating, the leaders' refusal to give up or give in and reciprocate with hostility or obvious frustration communicates clearly to clients that no matter what they do or how withdrawn they are, the group will progress and continue.

On the other hand, leaders can do only so much with a group if the group members are withdrawn and not talking. In these situations, it is helpful to be able to read the clients' minds. It is sometimes a good idea for the leaders to have a dialogue (out loud) with one another, trying to figure out the problem. Although over time the group members should develop the ability to resolve group stalemates with the leaders via problem solving, at the beginning progress is usually not visible. It is absolutely essential in these situations that leaders *not* let their own judgments and hostile interpretations have free rein. Compassion and empathy are essential.

Member versus Member. Not infrequently, there is conflict between individual members in a skills training group. In my experience, encouraging group members to discuss their problems with one another openly in group almost always results in disaster. Again, borderline clients, at least at their most dysfunctional, simply cannot tolerate criticism in a group setting; thus, member-to-member problems need to be dealt with privately until the collective ability to solve problems publicly is increased. In private interactions with a group member who is distressed (before or after a session or during a break), a leader's primary role is to soothe the distressed member and to explain the offending member in a sympathetic manner. If criticisms or member-to-member conflicts arise during a session, a leader's best strategy is to serve as the third point or fulcrum. Rather than suggesting that the conflicting members talk with one another to resolve their differences or hurt feelings, the leader should publicly defend the offending member while simultaneously empathizing with the offended member.

If the conflict is over procedural issues, problem solving can go forward in the group session. For example, a conflict arose in one of our skills training groups between one member's need for the window curtains to be closed and other group members' need for the curtains to be open. Such conflicts should be mediated by a group leader but can be discussed in group sessions. Many such conflicts will arise over the course of the year. A leader's role in these is somewhat like a parent's or teacher's role with a group of problem children. The sensitivities of each individual member must be respected; a leader must resist the tendency at times to sacrifice one member for the good of the whole.

Leader versus Leader. Perhaps the most damaging conflict in conducting DBT group skills training is that which can arise between the two group leaders. Smooth coordination can be especially difficult when the leaders have different theoretical perspectives, have different views of how psychotherapy groups should be conducted, or wish for a different role in the skills training than the role assigned. These issues need to be resolved outside of the skills training sessions, preferably before the first session. When conflicts arise in sessions, the usual procedure is for the coleader to defer to the primary leader during the session and argue his or her case afterwards.

A problem arises when the coleader is better tuned in both to group members and to the unfolding process than the primary leaders. This is a situation where the DBT supervision/consultation team can be quite useful. No matter what the difference in experience between leaders may be, it is important for them not to fall into the trap of who is "right" and who is "wrong." Not only is this approach dialectically flawed, but it is rarely useful in resolving a conflict.

A related situation that sometimes occurs is that when one group leader is absent, group members complain about the absent leader to the other leader. How should the leader who is present react? The most important thing is not to become split off from the absent leader. The same strategy used when an absent member is being discussed should be employed. That is, the present leader should portray the absent leader in a sympathetic light, while simultaneously validating the concerns of the members present. It is a tricky line to walk, but essential nonetheless.

Relationship Generalization

The principles of relationship generalization in DBT skills training are the same as those in DBT individual psychotherapy. Leaders must be vigilant in noticing when interpersonal relationships within the group are similar to problems individuals are having outside of group sessions. A number of typical problems show up in group skills training. Borderline individuals' exquisite sensitivity to criticism and the rapid onset of extreme shame almost always create problems; the public nature of the group setting simply exacerbates these problems. In addition, the group setting is often reminiscent of family interactions. Problems that individuals have with their families are likely to show up in the group. Many members have problems in coping with authority figures, especially when the authority figures are telling them what to do. Therefore, at least some patients will have problems with doing homework practice. At other times, problems concern whether individual members will admit to progress. The problems of borderline individuals in regard to competence and the appearance of competence are discussed extensively in Chapters 3 and 10 of the text.

The inability of many borderline individuals to put personal problems on a shelf, so to speak, and attend to the skills training material is quite similar to their difficulties outside of skills training in work or school settings. Their inability to remember to practice skills (or to get themselves to practice even when they do remember), and then to punish or berate themselves in a judgmental fashion, is indicative of their general difficulties with self-management. Their tendency to withdraw

emotionally and become silent when any conflict occurs during group sessions is typical of their difficulties in dealing with conflict outside of the group. An often unstated, but particularly difficult, problem of many group members is their inability to shut themselves off emotionally from other group members' pain. Consequent exacerbation of their own painful emotions can result in either panic attacks, hostile behavior, or complete emotional withdrawal. As can be seen from just this partial list, skills training in a group setting can be counted on to bring up many of the everyday problems that borderline individuals have.

Using relationship generalization strategies in group skills training sessions, however, can be quite tricky. The basic idea is to help a member see how her everyday problems are showing up within the skills training group, without at the same time invalidating her real problems with the group or with specific members. It is important that leaders not be overinclined to attribute all within-therapy problems to prior problems that members have rather than to inadequacies in the group format or to the leaders' application of the treatment.

Borderline client's difficulties in accepting negative feedback or implied criticism suggest that leaders must be extremely sensitive in applying the relationship generalization strategies. In my own experience, the best way to do this is to take an individual problem, make it into a universal problem, and then discuss it in that context. The astute group member may figure out that she is the one is being talked to, but still it is not a public humiliation.

The first step in relationship generalization is to relate the within-session relationship problem to general problems that need work both in and out of the skills training group. Just making this connection (an insight strategy; see Chapter 9 of the text) can sometimes be therapeutic. The next step is to use problem-solving strategies to develop alternative response patterns for members to try. The key in relationship generalization, in skills training as in psychotherapy, is to plan for rather than to assume generalization. Planning, at a minimum, requires discussion with the group members. The discussion should also include developing homework in which clients can practice applying new skills to everyday situations. Since this is the essential idea undergirding skills training and homework practice anyway, relationship generalization is especially compatible with DBT skills training.

The next five chapters present the outline (Chapter 6) and content (Chapters 7–10) of the four skills training modules. The handouts and homework sheets to be given to skills training clients are all together at the end of the book to facilitate efficient photocopying.

6

Session-by-Session Outlines for Psychosocial Skills Training

Instructional material in skills training, especially in a group context should be presented by the skills trainers at a pace adapted to the level of understanding of the clients. At periodic intervals during each skills training session, participants should be asked "comprehension" questions designed to test whether they understand key points being communicated. Misunderstood material should be reviewed. Since the pace of each session will differ, as will the overall pace for particular individuals or groups, instructional content is not divided into segments for particular sessions. In order to facilitate the coverage of all of the material by the end of the time scheduled for the particular module, however, the skills training leaders should construct lesson plans for each session and should attempt to cover the designated material during the session time allotted.

In my experience, the first time therapists teach these skill modules the amount of material feels overwhelming, and the therapists tend to spend too much time on early parts of a module and then have too little time later to cover other material that may be more important. However, what actually is important will necessarily vary with different individuals or groups, depending on their experience and skill levels. Therefore, the best strategy the first time through is to cut each module arbitrarily into sections corresponding to the exact number of weeks you have and try to get through as much of each section as possible. That experience will dictate how to time the modules the second time, and so on. When I teach therapists how to do DBT skills training, I usually recommend that trainers first teach the material in the skills modules in the order given in this manual. After the first run-through, modifications in content and order can be made to better suit the particular situation.

One goal of the skills training sessions is to impart information about particular coping strategies to participants. A second, equally important goal is to elicit from the participants rules and strategies for effective coping that they have learned in the particular situations they encounter. Thus, skills training should be taught so that the instructional material is augmented as a result of each discussion. Participants should be encouraged to take notes and to expand the handout materials furnished during sessions with their own and other participants' ideas. Whenever a particularly good strategy is presented in a session, all should be instructed to write it down in the appropriate space on their handouts (including the skills training leaders). The strategy should then be included in practice and review, just as are strategies presented initially by the leaders.

When therapists are using these guidelines for the first time, it can be helpful to go through them first and highlight key points to be covered. I have tried to do this as well by using bold face type for key topics. For the first session in each module, when therapists are presenting or reviewing the general rationale of skills training, they can use the outline in this chapter as a guide in actually conducting the session. For the remaining chapters, the content outlines in Chapters 7–10 will be needed.

Session 1: Orientation to Skills Training

In a group context, the purpose of the first session is to introduce members to one another and to the skills training leaders; to orient members to the structural aspects of the therapy (e.g., format, rules, meeting times);

and to orient them to the leaders' theoretical approach to BPD and goals for the class. This session is repeated at the beginning of each 8-week module. However, after the first orientation class, reorientation may be abbreviated if there are no new members starting the new module. If there are new members, the leaders should try to get old members to conduct as much of the orientation as possible. In either case, if orientation is concluded before the session ends, the leaders should proceed to the material for Session 2 (core mindfulness skills).

Material in this session covering format, timing, fees, rules, use of the telephone, and so on should be changed to reflect particular circumstances. Thus, this section provides an outline of topics to be covered, but the content of at least some of the topics can be easily modified. (If a therapist is teaching skills individually, most of the information will be the same. The structured aspects, however, will be quite different, since many concern relationships among group members and between group members and leaders.)

I. **Review consent forms** for therapy. Be sure consent forms are signed. Fill out relevant research and/or assessment forms.

II. Ask each participant to **introduce** herself with her name and a brief statement of why she is here (and, for a previous participant, how long she has been in treatment program). Leaders: Introduce yourselves and give information about yourselves and why you are leading skills training.

III. Give **general goals.**

  A. Therapy/skills training for clients.

  B. Income, other goals of therapists.

  C. Training of therapists (coleaders) (if applicable).

  D. Research (if applicable).

IV. Review General Handout I: Goals of Skills Training

  A. **General goal of skills training:** To learn and refine skills in changing behavioral, emotional, and thinking patterns associated with problems in living that are causing misery and distress.

  B. **Specific goals:** Discuss relationship of borderline characteristics to specific skills training modules. (See Chapter 5 of the text and Chapter 1 of this manual for discussions of this point.) Get feedback from participants on

whether or not each behavioral pattern is characteristic of them.

1. **Interpersonal chaos:** Discuss intense, unstable relationships; trouble maintaining relationships; panic, anxiety, and dread over relationships ending; frantic attempts to avoid abandonment.

   Interpersonal effectiveness training focuses on this characteristic of BPD. However, it focuses specifically on learning to deal with conflict situations, to get what one wants and needs, and to say no to unwanted requests and demands. It focuses specifically on doing this in a manner that maintains self-respect and others' liking and/or respect. Thus, it does not focus on all aspects of relationships.

2. **Labile affect,** moods, emotions: Discuss extreme emotional sensitivity, ups and downs, moodiness, intense emotional reactions; chronic depression; problems with anger (either overcontrolled or undercontrolled).

   Emotion regulation training focuses on enhancing control of emotions, even though *complete* emotional control cannot be achieved. Explain: "To a certain extent we are who we are, and emotionality is part of us. But we can get more control and perhaps can learn to modulate some emotions to be a bit more mellow."

3. **Impulsiveness:** Discuss problems with alcohol, drugs, eating, spending, sex, fast driving, etc. Also, discuss parasuicidal behavior (see Chapter 1 of the text for definition), suicide threats.

   Distress tolerance training focuses on learning to tolerate distress. Discuss the connection between inability to tolerate distress and impulsive behavior which very often functions to reduce intolerable distress.

4. **Confusion about self, cognitive dysregulation:** Discuss problems experiencing or identifying a self; a pervasive sense of emptiness; problems in maintaining one's own feelings, opinions, decisions when around others. Also discuss brief, nonpsychotic cognitive disturbances (depersonalization, dissociation, delusions).

   Core mindfulness training focuses on learning to go within to find oneself and on learning to observe oneself.

C. Get feedback.

V. Discuss **format** of skills training.

   A. Describe **order** and **length** of modules.

   B. Describe **use of session time** (half for discussing homework practice, half for presenting new material).

   C. Make it clear that neither time nor format allows for discussion of personal problems unrelated to using behavioral skills. **Personal problems should be discussed with individual psychotherapist.** Note that this is not due to lack of compassion, but to need to use session time to teach coping skills.

   D. Discuss use of **telephone calls** to skills training leaders. Calls should only pertain to sessions (either missing a session or some other pertinent topic). Personal crises (including suicidal crises) should be discussed with individual psychotherapist, crisis clinic, emergency room, relatives, friends. Give phone numbers to contact group leaders.

VI. Review General Handout 2: Guidelines for Skills Training.

   A. Discuss and get each participant to agree to rules. (See Chapter 3 of this manual for a discussion of each of the rules.)

   B. Discuss any rules not on list.

   C. Discuss what an "excused" session is (e.g., session missed because of physical illness, family emergency, vacation out of town, wedding, funeral) and what an "unexcused" session is (e.g., session missed because of fatigue, bad mood, psychiatric hospitalization, solvable problem).

Session 2: Core Mindfulness Skills

   I. Discuss any **questions** from last week.

   II. **Introduce** new participants.

   A. **Review** DBT skills training rules. Have other participants explain guidelines to new ones.

III. Review diary cards and how to fill out.

   A. On the front of the card, **only the last column** (rating degree of behavioral skills practice) will be discussed in sessions. All other sections on front of card will be discussed during individual psychotherapy. Encourage those who have

non-DBT individual psychotherapists to discuss diary card and its contents with their individual therapists.

   The **entire back** of the card (pertaining to skills) will be discussed in sessions each week. **Tell clients to bring their card every week!**

   B. Degree of behavioral skills practice (front of diary card) is rated according to scale at bottom of card. Any adaptive, active problem solving is considered a skill. Thus, participants should rate their use of skills, including use of any and all coping skills not taught in class. Note that use of maladaptive problem solving (drinking, self-cutting, etc.) does not count as using skills.

   C. On back of diary card, participants should circle each skill each day if they make *any attempt* to practice the skill. Use this as an opportunity to discuss the role of self-monitoring, feedback, and reinforcement in behavior change. (See Chapter 9 of the text for a discussion of these points.)

   D. Discuss crucial importance of **practice** in learning and change.

   E. **Troubleshoot** problems in filling out diary cards. Engage in problem solving for difficulties that arise.

   F. Discuss **confidentiality of cards**, ways to keep confidential. Give out alternative cards with only acronyms, if necessary.[1] Suggest that participants not put real names on cards.

   IV. Introduce, discuss, and practice **core mindfulness skills** (see Chapter 7 of this manual).

   V. **Summarize** key points of content discussed during class.

   VI. Develop **practice commitments.**

   A. Go around and discuss with each person what she will practice during the coming week. Participants can choose a particular skill to practice across a wide array of situations, or they can pick a recurrent problem situation to practice in. In the latter case, the objective is to use a variety of skills in the problem situation.

   B. Make an effort to get each participant to agree to practice observing and describing during the first few weeks. Over subsequent modules, each person should focus some practice on each of the six mindfulness skills.

   C. **Troubleshoot** problems in implementing practice.

VII. Conduct session **wind-down.**

 A. Select one of the wind-down exercises described in Chapter 3 of this manual. During this session, instruct participants in how to do wind-down. Give rationale for using a wind-down.

 B. Suggest that participants bring tapes of favorite music to listen to at end of skills training sessions. Work out a scheme for rotating task.

Session 3–7: Specific Module Skills

 I. Discuss any **questions** from last week.

 II. Check in with **individuals who did not attend** last session.

 A. Discuss reasons for not attending session(s).

 B. Briefly review content of previous session. Have other participants briefly explain previous material to ones who were absent.

 III. **Review homework** practice.

 A. Go from person to person, asking each whether she practiced any new (or old) skills during the previous week. Use therapy-interfering behavior strategies (see Chapter 15 of text and Chapter 5 of this manual) if she did not practice. Use problem-solving strategies (see Chapter 9 of text and Chapter 5 of this manual) if she practiced but couldn't implement skills, or if she did implement them but they did not help. Blend confrontation, shaping, and validation. Highlight and reinforce success.

 B. Be alert to a person's always using the same skill and not practicing any new skills. The objective here is for everyone to develop the ability to implement each skill. If once a person has a skill capability, she then chooses never to use it in her daily life, this is OK.

 IV. Take a midpoint **break** (after first hour or so).

 V. Present, discuss, and practice **skills content for specific module** (see Chapters 7–10 of this manual).

 VI. **Summarize** content presented.

 VII. Develop **practice commitments.**

 A. Go around and discuss with each person what she will practice during the coming week. Participants can choose a particular skill to practice across a wide array of situations, or they can pick a recurrent problem situation to practice in. In the latter case, the objective is to use a variety of skills in the problem situation.

 B. Check that practice plans and agreements are in line with the homework sheets given out for that particular session.

 C. **Troubleshoot** problems in implementing practice.

 VIII. Conduct session **wind-down.**

Session 8: Last Session

 I–III. First hour: Same as sessions 3–7.

 IV. Take a midpoint **break.**

 V. **Review skills** that have been taught during **this module.**

 VI. Review **skills from previous modules.**

 A. Briefly review essential skills in previous modules if any members have been in those modules.

 B. Ask participants to supplement review by listing any skills from previous modules that they found especially helpful or that they need more practice in.

 VII. **Discuss pros and cons,** uses and misuses, helpfulness and nonhelpfulness of different skills, including skills from previous modules. Compare notes on use among participants.

 VIII. Discuss **skill generalization** across situations and contexts of participants' lives.

 IX. Say **good-bye** to any individuals leaving skills training. Discuss termination issues. (See Chapter 4 of this manual and Chapter 14 of the text for further discussion of termination.)

 X. Conduct session and module **wind-down.** During last class of each module, wind-down should consist of observations about the entire 8-week series of classes. Focus on observations about how the weeks went, how sessions went, and how participants felt and feel about the module.

Note

 1. Some individuals do not want to use diary cards that can be understood by anyone else if they are found. In these instances, revised diary cards that use acronyms instead of the names of skills and other items can be employed. Alternatively, a client can use a number or pseudonym instead of her real name on the cards.

7

Core Mindfulness Skills

Mindfulness skills are central to DBT (hence the label "core" mindfulness skills). They are the first skills taught and are listed on the diary cards that clients fill out every week. These are the only skills that are highlighted the entire year; they are reviewed at the beginning of each of the other three skill modules. The skills are psychological and behavioral versions of meditation practices from Eastern spiritual training. I have drawn most heavily from the practice of Zen, but the skills are compatible with most Western contemplative and Eastern meditation practices.

In DBT, three primary states of mind are presented: "reasonable mind," "emotion mind," and "wise mind." A person is in "reasonable mind" when she is approaching knowledge intellectually, is thinking rationally and logically, attends to empirical facts, is planful in her behavior, focuses her attention, and is "cool" in her approach to problems. The person is in "emotion mind" when her thinking and behavior are controlled primarily by her current emotional state. In "emotion mind," cognitions are "hot"; reasonable, logical thinking is difficult; facts are amplified or distorted to be congruent with current affect; and the energy of behavior is also congruent with the current emotional state. "Wise mind" is the integration of "emotion mind" and "reasonable mind," as I have noted in Chapter 5 of this manual. It also and goes beyond them: "Wise mind" adds intuitive knowing to emotional experiencing and logical analysis.

Mindfulness skills are the vehicles for balancing "emotion mind" and "reasonable mind" to achieve "wise mind." There are three "what" skills (observing, describing, and participating) and three "how" skills (taking a nonjudgmental stance, focusing on one thing in the moment, and being effective).

Mindfulness "What" Skills

The mindfulness "what" skills include learning to observe, to describe, and to participate. The goal is to develop a lifestyle of participating with awareness; an assumption of DBT is that participation without awareness is a characteristic of impulsive and mood dependent behaviors. Generally, observing and describing one's own behavioral responses are only necessary when new behavior is being learned, there is some sort of problem, or a change is necessary. For example, beginning piano players pay close attention to the location of their hands and fingers, and may either count beats out loud or name the keys and chords they are playing. As skill improves, however, such observing and describing cease. But if a habitual mistake is made after a piece is learned, the player may have to revert to observing and describing until a new pattern has been learned. Learning to drive a stick-shift car, to dance, and to type are other familiar examples of this principle.

The first "what" skill is observing—that is, attending to events, emotions, and other behavioral responses, without *necessarily* trying to terminate them when painful or prolong them when pleasant. What the client learns here is to allow herself to experience with awareness, in the moment, whatever is happening, rather than leaving a situation or trying to terminate an emotion. Generally, the ability to attend to events requires a corresponding ability to step back from the event. Observing an event is separate or different from the event itself. Observing walking and walking are two different responses; observing thinking and thinking are two different responses; observing one's own heartbeat and the heart's beating are two different responses. This focus on "experiencing the moment" is based on Eastern psychological approaches, as well as on Western notions of nonreinforced exposure as a method of extinguishing automatic avoidance and fear responses.

A second mindfulness "what" skill is that of describing events and personal responses in words. The ability to apply verbal labels to behavioral and environmental events is essential for both communication and self-control. Learning to describe requires that a person learn not to take emotions and thoughts literally—that is, as literal reflections of environmental events. For example, feeling afraid does not necessarily mean that a situation is threatening to life or welfare. Many people, including borderline individuals, confuse emotional responses with precipitating events. Physical components of fear ("I feel my stomach muscles tightening, my throat constricting") may be confused with perceptions of the environment ("I am starting an exam in school") to produce a dysfunctional thought ("I am going to fail the exam"). Thoughts are often taken literally; that is, thoughts ("I feel unloved") are confused with facts ("I am unloved"). One of the principal aims of cognitive therapy is to test the association of thoughts with their corresponding environmental events.

The third mindfulness "what" skill is the ability to participate without self-consciousness. A person who is participating is entering completely into the activities of the current moment, without separating herself from ongoing events and interactions. The quality of action is spontaneous; the interaction between the individual and the environment is smooth and based in some part on habit. Participating can, of course, be mindless. We have all had the experience of driving a complicated path to home as we concentrated on something else, arriving home without any awareness whatsoever of how we got there. But it can also be mindful. A good example of mindful participating is that of the skillful athlete who responds flexibly but smoothly to the demands of the task with alertness and awareness, but not with self-consciousness. Mindlessness is participating without attention to the task; mindfulness is participating with attention.

Mindfulness "How" Skills

The other three mindfulness skills have to do with *how* one attends, describes, and participates; they include taking a nonjudgmental stance, focusing on one thing in the moment, and being effective (doing what works). As taught in DBT, taking a nonjudgmental stance means just that—taking a nonevaluative approach, judging something as neither good nor bad. It does not mean going from a negative judgment to a positive judgment.

Although borderline individuals tend to judge both themselves and others in either excessively positive terms (idealization) or excessively negative terms (devaluation), the position here is not that they should be more balanced in their judgments, but rather that judging should in most instances be dropped altogether. This is a very subtle point but a very important one. The problem with judging is that, for instance, a person who can be "worthwhile" can always become "worthless." Instead, DBT stresses a focus on the consequences of behavior and events. For example, a person's behavior may lead to painful consequences for herself or for others, or the outcome of events may be destructive. A nonjudgmental approach observes these consequences, and may suggest changing the behaviors or events, but would not necessarily add a label of "bad" to them.

Mindfulness in its totality has to do with the quality of awareness that a person brings to activities. The second "how" is to learn to focus the mind and awareness in the current moment's activity, rather than splitting attention among several activities or between a current activity and thinking about something else. Achieving such a focus requires control of attention, a capability that most borderline individuals lack. Often borderline clients are distracted by thoughts and images of the past, worries about the future, ruminative thoughts about troubles, or current negative moods. They are sometimes unable to put their troubles away and focus attention on the task at hand. When they do become involved in a task, their attention is often divided. This problem is readily observable in their difficulties in attending to skills training sessions. The clients need to learn how to focus their attention on one task or activity at a time, engaging in it with alertness, awareness, and wakefulness.

The third "how" goal, being effective, is directed at reducing the client's tendency at times to be more concerned with what is "right" than with doing what is actually needed or called for in a particular situation. Effectiveness is the opposite of "cutting off your nose to spite your face." As our clients often say, it is "playing the game" or "doing what works." From an Eastern meditation perspective, focusing on effectiveness is "using skillful means." The inability to let go of "being right" in favor of achieving goals is, of course, related to borderline individuals' experiences with invalidating environments. A central issue for many clients is whether they can indeed trust their own perceptions, judgments, and decisions—that is, whether they can expect their own actions to be correct or "right." However, taken to an extreme, an emphasis on principle over outcome can often result in the clients' being disappointed or alienating others. In the end, we all have to "give in" some of the time. Borderline clients at times find it much easier to give up being right for being effective when it is viewed as a skillful response rather than as a "giving in."

Homework Practice

In contrast to the other three modules, the mindfulness skills module does not have any homework practice sheets. Clients are simply asked to practice the skills learned so far during every week. As noted earlier, all of the mindfulness skills are listed on the back of the diary cards; members should be instructed to circle each skill each day that they make any attempt to practice their skills. If individual clients wish to, they can keep a written diary of their efforts and bring their notes to skills training sessions.

Content Outline

I. **Orient** clients to skills to be learned in this module and the rationale for their importance.
   A. **Explain focus of core mindfulness skills:** "Learning to be in control of your own mind, instead of letting your mind be in control of you."

Discussion Point: To a certain extent, being in control of one's mind is actually learning to be in control of attention processes—that is, what one pays attention to and how long one pays attention to it. Draw from participants examples of how their inability to control their attention creates problems. Examples may include inability to stop thinking about things, (e.g., the past, the future, current emotional pain or hurt, physical pain); inability to concentrate on a task when it is important to do so; inability to focus on another person or to stay on a task because of distraction.

   B. Mindfulness skills requires **practice, practice, practice.**

Lecture Point: Relate learning to take control of one's mind to Western and Eastern traditions of meditation developed over thousands of years. All rely on practice. Relate to yoga master's ability to withstand pain, walk on red-hot coals, etc.

Note to Leaders: Sometimes individuals will be put off by references to Eastern meditation practice. You need to be very sensitive to this point. You can either divorce meditation from any religion or relate it to all religions. (1) Meditation is now commonly used in the treatment of chronic physical pain and stress management programs, and is increasingly being used in treatment of emotional disorders. Thus, meditation can be practiced outside of any spiritual or religious context. (2) Eastern meditation practice is very similar to Chris-

tian contemplative prayer, Jewish mystical tradition, and forms of prayer taught in other religions.

Discussion Point: Discuss with participants the crucial importance of behavioral practice in learning any new skill. Behavioral practice includes practicing control of one's mind, attention, overt behavior, body, and emotions. Draw from participants their beliefs about the necessity of practice in learning: "Can you learn without practice?"

II. Review Mindfulness Handout 1: Taking Hold of Your Mind: States of Mind.

   A. **Reasonable mind.** Explain: "This is your rational, thinking, logical mind. It is that part of you that plans and evaluates things logically. It is your cool part."

Lecture Point: Reasonable mind can be very beneficial. Without it, people could not build homes, roads, or cities; they could not follow instructions; they could not solve logical problems, do science, or run meetings.

Lecture Point: Reasonable mind is easier when people feel good, and much harder when they don't.

Discussion Point: When other people say that "if you could just think straight you would be all right," they mean that "if you could be in reasonable mind you would do OK." Elicit from participants times other people have said or implied that if they would just not distort, exaggerate, or misperceive things, they would have far fewer problems. How many times have participants said the same thing to themselves? Isn't there some truth to these positions?

   B. **Emotion mind.** Explain: "You are in emotion mind when your emotions are in control—when they influence and control your thinking and your behavior."

Lecture Point: Emotion mind can be very beneficial. Intense love fills history books as motivation for relationships. Intense love (or intense hate) has fueled wars. Intense devotion or desire motivates staying with very hard tasks, sacrificing oneself for others (e.g., mothers running through fires for their children).

Lecture Point: A certain amount of emotion mind is desirable. Borderline individuals have more than most; they are the "dramatic" folks of the world and will always be so. People high in emotion mind are often passionate about people, causes, beliefs, etc.

Lecture Point: Problems with emotion mind occur when the results are positive in the short term but negative in the long term, or when the experience itself is very painful, or leads to other painful states and events (e.g., anxiety and depression can be painful in themselves).

Lecture Point: Emotion mind is exacerbated by (1) illness; (2) sleep deprivation, tiredness; (3) drugs, alcohol; (4) hunger, bloating, overeating, poor nutrition; (5) environmental stress (too many demands); and (6) environmental threats. Elicit other factors from participants.

Discussion Point: Discuss pros and cons of both types of mind. Draw from participants their experience of reasonable mind and of emotion mind.

C. **Wise mind.** Explain: "Wise mind is the integration of emotion mind and reasonable mind. You cannot overcome emotion mind with reasonable mind. Nor can you create emotions with reasonableness. You must go within and integrate the two."

Note to Leaders: You need not cover each of these points every time through; give just enough to get your point across. You will be covering this section many times. Expand on your points a bit more each time through. (See Chapter 7 of the text for a fuller discussion of wise mind.)

Lecture Point: Wise mind is that part of each person that can know and experience truth. It is where the person knows something to be true or valid. It is almost always quiet; it has a certain peace. It is where the person knows something in a centered way.

Lecture Point: Wisdom, wise mind, or wise knowing depends upon integration of all ways of knowing something: knowing by observing, knowing by analyzing logically, knowing by what we experience in our bodies (kinetic and sensory experience), knowing by what we do, and knowing by intuition (May, 1982).

Lecture Point: Wise mind is similar to intuition. (Or, perhaps, intuition is part of wise mind.) It is knowing that is more than reasoning and more than what is observed directly. It has qualities of direct experience; immediate knowing; understanding the meaning, significance, or truth of an event without having to analyze it intellectually (Deikman, 1982); and "feelings of deepening coherence" (Polanyi, 1958).

Lecture Point: Everyone has wise mind; some simply have never experienced it. Also, no one is in wise mind all the time.

Discussion Point: Get feedback from participants on their own experiences of wise mind.

Note to Leaders: Clients will sometimes say that they don't have wise mind. You must cheerlead here. Believe in clients' abilities to find wise mind. Wise mind is like having a heart; everyone has one, whether they experience it or not. Use the "well" analogy below.

Lecture Point: Explain: "Wise mind is like a deep well in the ground. The water at the bottom of the well, the entire underground ocean is wise mind. But on the way down there are often trap doors that impede progress. Sometimes the trap doors are so cleverly built that you actually believe that there is no water at the bottom of the well. The trap door may look like the bottom of the well. Perhaps it is locked and you need a key. Perhaps it is nailed shut and you need a hammer, or it is glued shut and you need a chisel."

Discussion Point: Elicit examples from participants. For example, sometimes a person may reach wisdom only when suddenly confronted by another person. Or someone else may say something insightful that unlocks an inner door.

Lecture Point: Wise mind is sometimes experienced in the center of the body (the belly), or in the center of the head, or between the eyes. Sometimes a person can find it by following the breath in and out.

Practice Exercise: Have participants go into themselves and experience wise mind. Explain: "Finding wise mind is like riding a bike; you can only learn it by experience." Instruct them to follow their breath (attend to their breath coming in and out) as they breathe naturally and deeply, and after some time to try to let their attention settle into their center, at the bottom of their inhalation. That very centered point is wise mind. Have participants share their experiences.

Discussion Point: Wise mind may be the calm that follows the storm—an experience immediately following a crisis or enormous chaos. It is suddenly getting to the heart of a matter, seeing or knowing something directly and clearly. It is grasping the whole picture when before only parts were understood. It is "feeling" the right choice in a dilemma, when the feeling comes from deep within rather from a current emotional state. Elicit similar experiences and other examples from participants.

D. **Emotion mind versus wise mind: how to know the difference.**

Lecture Point: Emotion mind and wise mind both have a quality of "feeling" something to be the case. The intensity of emotions can generate experiences of certainty that mimic the stable, cool certainty of wisdom. Continue the analogy above: "After a heavy rain, water can collect on a trap door within the well. You may then confuse the still water on the trap door with the deep ocean at the bottom of the well."

Discussion Point: There is no simple solution here. Suggest: "If intense emotion is obvious, suspect emotion mind. Give it time; if certainty remains, especially when you are feeling calm and secure, suspect wise mind." Ask participants for other ideas on how to tell the difference.

III. Review Mindfulness Handout 2: Taking Hold of Your Mind: "What" Skills.

A. Describe two types of mindfulness skills: (1) **"what" skills** (i.e., what to do) and (2) **"how" skills** (i.e., how to do it).

B. With respect to "what" skills, it is very important to point out that a person can only do one thing at a time—observe, or describe, or participate, but not all three at once. In contrast, the "how" skills can be applied all at once.

C. **Observing.** Explain: "Observing is sensing or experiencing without describing or labeling the experience. It is noticing or attending to something."

Practice Exercises: Have participants try some of the following.

1. "Experience your fanny on the chair."
2. "Experience your hand on a cool surface (e.g., a table or chair) or a warm surface (e.g., your other hand)."
3. "Attend to and try to sense your stomach, your shoulders."
4. "Stroke just above your upper lip, then stop stroking and notice how long it takes before you can't sense your upper lip any longer."
5. " 'Watch' in your mind the first two thoughts that come in."
6. "Imagine that your mind is a conveyor belt, and that thoughts and/or feelings are coming down the belt. Put each thought and/or feeling in a box near the belt."
7. "Imagine that your mind is the sky and thoughts, sensations and/or feelings are clouds. Gently notice each cloud as it drifts by (or scurries by)."
8. "If you find yourself describing thoughts, sensations, or feelings, 'step back', in your mind so to speak, and observe your describing."
9. "If you find yourself distracted, observe that; observe yourself as you become aware that you were distracted."

Note to Leaders: It is essential to help clients observe in a nonattached way. Thus, whatever happens in their minds is "grist for the mill," so to speak. No matter what they do, they can just "step back" and observe. Get feedback. Work with clients until they get the idea of observing. Check how long each person can observe. It is common to have to start and restart many times in the course of 1 or 2 minutes.

Lecture Point: Remind participants to step back within themselves, not outside of themselves to observe. Observing is not dissociating. If an individual has difficulty staying inside instead of going outside of herself, suggest that she try the following: "Imagine that the place you go outside of yourself is a flower. The flower is connected to your center by a long stem. The center is the root of the flower. Imagine coming down the stem to the root. Do this each time."

D. **Describing.** Explain: "Describing is using words to represent what you observe."

Lecture Point: Observing is like sensing; there are no words. Observing is noticing and attending. Describing is a reaction to observing; it is labeling what is observed.

Discussion Point: Discuss the difference between describing and observing. Again, observing is like sensing without words. Describing is using words or thoughts to label what is observed.

Discussion Point: Discuss how describing a thought as a thought requires one to notice that it is a thought instead of a fact. Give examples of the differences between thinking "I am a jerk" and being a jerk. Get feedback. Get lots of examples. It is crucial that clients get this distinction.

Practice Exercise: Have participants practice observing thoughts and labeling them as thoughts. Suggest labeling them into categories (e.g., "thoughts about myself," "thoughts about others," etc.) Use the conveyor belt exercise above, but this time as thoughts and feelings come down the belt, have participants sort them into categories: "For example, you could have one box for thoughts (of any sort), one box for sensations in your body, one box for urges to do something (for example, urges to stop)."

Discussion Point: Discuss the difference between describing and judging. Judging is labeling something in an evaluative way. Describing is "just the facts."

E. **Participating.** Explain: "Participating is entering wholly into an activity, becoming one with the activity. It is throwing yourself into something. It is spontaneous behavior to a certain extent, although you can also do it mindfully."

Discussion Point: Note that participating is the ultimate goal. The only reason we observe and describe is to understand and improve things. Share examples of participating (e.g., driving a car): "When we switch cars to one with a different way of driving or if we go to England and have to drive on the left side of the road, we suddenly need to stop and observe and describe." Gather other examples from clients.

F. **Discuss relationship of the three skills.** Discuss with clients which "what" skill (observing, describing, participating) is their strength and which is their weakness. The one they have most difficulty with is the one to practice the most.

IV. Review Mindfulness Handout 3: Taking Hold of Your Mind: "How" Skills.

A. **Nonjudgmentally.** The goal here is to take a nonjudgmental stance when observing, describing, and participating. Judging is any labeling or evaluating of something as good or bad, as valuable or not, as worthwhile or worthless. The essence of it is the valuing of things as more or less "good" or "bad." An important mindfulness skill is *not* judging things in this manner.

Lecture Point: Point out the difference between judging what a person does, which is applying a label of "good" or "bad," and describing the consequences of what a person does. Consequences may be painful, destructive, or harmful. A person who stops judging can still observe or predict consequences. Sometimes judging is a shorthand way of describing consequences. For example, saying "This piece of meat is bad" is a shorthand way of saying "It is filled with bacteria and may make you sick if you eat it."

Discussion Point: Get examples of the difference between judging and noticing consequences: "Your behavior is terrible" versus "Your behavior is hurting me" or "What you are doing is going to result in my getting hurt"; "I am stupid (and bad)" versus "I missed my appointment for the third time and this is going to get me in trouble with my friends if I don't change."

Lecture Point: Point out how judging is sometimes a shorthand way of comparing things to a standard; in this case, judging gives information. For example, saying that a tomato is "bad" may mean that it is not like a fresh tomato. Or judging may be a shorthand way of stating a preference. Saying that a room looks "bad" or a book was "terrible" is based on a personal preference in decorating or in reading material (or, sometimes on a personal or community standard for how rooms should look or how books should be written). The problem is that over time, people forget that judging is shorthand and begin to take it literally as a statement of fact.

Discussion Point: Participants may believe that if people are saying something or someone is not "bad," then they must be saying it is "good," and vice versa. This is true only if people have the dichotomy "good–bad" in their minds in the first place and use that way of thinking to describe things. But thinking of things in terms of "good" and "bad" can be very harmful, and it is not necessary. Elicit from participants all the times others have applied judgments to them when they felt what they were doing, thinking, or feeling was neither good nor bad.

Discussion Point: Judging is often a way of getting out of responsibility. Explain: "If I don't like what other people are doing and want them to stop it, I can say, 'That is bad,' and don't have to own up to the fact that the real reason they should stop what they are doing is that I (and maybe everyone else too) don't like it, don't believe in it, or don't want the consequences." Elicit from participants times when others have tried to control their behavior by stating judgments as facts. Get examples of when they have tried that with someone else. Leaders: Give your own examples here.

Note to Leaders: Borderline individuals will frequently believe that there really is a "good" and a "bad." You need to be dialectical here and search for a synthesis of different points of view. Do not expect clients to throw out judgments without a fight! Expect clients to bring up Hitler (or, more rarely, sexual abuse) as an example of "bad" with a capital B. Thus, the next lecture point is important: Judgments have their place. Letting go of judging is an idea that will grow over time. Don't force it at the beginning. You can usually get more mileage out of focusing first on reducing self-judgments. (See Chapter 7 in the text for a more extensive discussion of these points.)

Lecture Point: Some people are paid to compare things to standards or to predict consequences—that is, to judge. Teachers give grades, grocers put out "good" food or produce and discard "bad" food. The word "good" is also used to give children and adults feedback about their behavior so they will know what to keep doing and what to stop. So one thing to remember is "Don't judge judging." It is essential at times. But most people overdo it, especially in judging themselves.

Discussion Point: Discuss the difference between a judgment and a statement of fact. A statement of fact may seem to be a judgment because the fact is simultaneously being judged. For instance, "I am fat" may simply be a statement of fact. But if one adds (in thoughts, implication, or tone of voice) that the idea being fat is bad or unattractive, then a judgment is added. A favorite judgmental word of clients I work with is "stupid," as in "I did a stupid thing," "I am stupid," or "What a stupid thing to say." Judgments often masquerade as statements of fact, so they can be hard to catch. Mental health professionals are very good at this sometimes. I once had a therapist try to convince me that calling a patient narcissistic (for saying she felt more "real" when she was around me) was not a judgmental statement. Get other examples.

B. **One-mindfully.** The goal here is to focus on one thing in the moment. Explain the process of doing one thing at a time with awareness. Emphasize focusing attention on only *one* activity or thing at a time, bringing the whole person to bear on a task or activity.

Lecture Point: This is the opposite of how people usually like to operate. Explain: "Most of us think that if we do several things at once we will accomplish more; this is not true. However, this does not mean that you cannot switch from one thing to another and back. The trick is to have your mind completely on what you are doing at the moment. This refers to both mental and physical activities."

Discussion Point: Discuss an example of doing two things at once, such as sitting in skills training and thinking about the past or worrying about the future. Explain: "A mindfulness perspective would suggest that if you are going to think about the past, you should devote your full attention to it. If you are going to worry about the future, devote your full attention to it. If you are going to attend class, devote your full attention to it." Get participants to come up with other examples (e.g., watching TV or reading while eating dinner).

Lecture Point: The notion of "worrying when you are worrying" is very similar to a very effective therapy for chronic worriers, developed by Thomas Borkovec (Borkovec & Inz, 1990). The essence of the therapy is setting aside 30 minutes each day to worry. Explain: "You go to the same place each day and try to spend the whole time worrying. During the rest of the day, you banish worries from your mind, reminding yourself that you will attend to that particular worry during your worry time. There is a similar technique for fighting insomnia: writing down all the things you need to remember for the next day before you go to sleep, so you won't have to wake up to think about them."

Lecture Point: Focusing on one thing in the moment does not mean that one cannot do complex tasks requiring many simultaneous activities. But it does mean that whatever one does, one should attend fully to it. Thus, the essence of the idea is acting with undivided attention. The opposites are mindlessness (i.e., automatic behaviors without awareness) and distracted behavior (i.e., doing one thing while thinking about or attending to another).

C. **Effectively.** The goal here is to focus on being effective—to focus on doing what works, rather than what is "right" versus "wrong" or "fair" versus "unfair." Generally, it is the opposite of "cutting off your nose to spite your face."

Lecture Point: Doing what works (or what is effective) requires knowing what one's goal or objective is. For instance, a person may want to get a raise at work, but she may also think that her supervisor should know without being told that she deserves one, so she refuses to ask for it. In this case, the person is putting being right over achieving her goal.

Lecture Point: Being effective requires knowing the actual situation and reacting to it, not to what one thinks *should* be the situation. For example, when driving on the freeway, people who drive more slowly are instructed by signs to drive in the right lane. People who tailgate slower drivers in the left lane (instead of just passing on the right) are acting as if all are prepared to follow the directions. All are not!

Lecture Point: Effectiveness is "playing by the rules." Playing by the rules is most important in situations where people are in a low-power position and what they want is important. A good example here is being an involuntary patient in a state hospital. Staff members make the rules about when a patient gets privileges. Right or wrong, they have the power, not the patients.

Discussion Point: Get examples of participants' "cutting off their noses" to make a point. Leaders: share examples of your own here as well—the more outrageous or humorous, the better.

Lecture Point: Effectiveness often means being "political" or savvy about people. It is taking people where they are (rather than where they "should" be) and going from there. Different people are like different cultures. What works in one culture may not work in another. Focusing on what's "right" instead of what works is like trying to impose one's own culture on another country when visiting.

Discussion Point: Get examples of when participants have imposed their own culture or views on others. When have others imposed in this way on participants?

Lecture Point: Effectiveness sometimes requires sacrificing principles to achieve a goal. In extreme situations (e.g., a concentration camp, where not playing by the rules would mean death), most people are willing to play by the rules even if they are not fair. In real life, this is sometimes very hard. It can be especially hard just when it is needed most, with people in authority positions.

D. Discuss with participants which "how" skill (taking a nonjudgmental stance, focusing on one thing in the moment, being effective) is their strength and which is their weakness. The one they have most difficulty with is the one to practice the most.

VI. **Summarize** states of mind, mindfulness "what" skills (observing, describing, participating), and mindfulness "how" skills (taking a nonjudgmental stance, focusing on one thing in the moment, being effective).

8

Interpersonal Effectiveness Skills

Goals of the Module

Interpersonal response patterns taught in DBT skills training are very similar to those taught in many assertiveness and interpersonal problem-solving classes. They include effective strategies for asking for what one needs, saying no, and coping with interpersonal conflict. "Effectiveness" here has to do with obtaining changes one wants, maintaining the relationship, and maintaining your self-respect. The particular behavioral patterns needed for social effectiveness are almost totally a function of a person's goals in a particular situational context. Thus, the ability to analyze a situation and to determine goals is crucial for interpersonal effectiveness. The first section of the interpersonal effectiveness module addresses this problem.

Borderline individuals frequently possess good interpersonal skills in a general sense. The problems arise in the application of these skills to specific situations. An individual may be able to describe effective behavioral sequences when discussing another person encountering a problematic situation, but may be completely incapable of generating or carrying out a similar behavioral sequence when analyzing her own situation. Usually, the problem is that belief patterns as well as uncontrollable emotional responses are inhibiting the application of the skills the person has.

One of the primary behavioral mistakes that borderline individuals make is premature termination of relationships. Such termination probably results from difficulties in all of the skill areas. Problems in distress tolerance make it difficult to tolerate fears, anxieties, or frustrations that are typical in conflictual situations. Problems in emotion regulation lead to inability to decrease chronic anger or frustration; inadequate interpersonal problem-solving skills make it difficult to turn

potential relationship conflicts into positive encounters. Problems with attending to the moment in a nonjudgmental fashion (i.e., problems with mindfulness) make it difficult either to assess personal wishes and goals or to assess what is needed to improve the situation. Interpersonal effectiveness skills are difficult to develop in a vacuum; perhaps more than any other set of skills, they depend on simultaneous improvement across all skill areas.

Borderline individuals frequently vacillate between avoidance of conflict and intense confrontation. Unfortunately, the choice of avoidance versus confrontation is usually based on an individual's emotional state rather than on the needs of the current situation. In general, skills training challenges clients' negative expectancies regarding their environment, their relationships, and themselves. In this module, the goal is to teach clients how to apply specific interpersonal problem-solving, social, and assertiveness skills to modify aversive environments and to obtain their goals in interpersonal encounters. The module focuses on situations where the objective is to change something (e.g., requesting someone to do something) or to resist changes someone else is trying to make (e.g., saying no). Thus, it is most properly considered a course in assertion, where the goal is for persons to assert their own wishes, goals, and opinions in a manner that causes other people to take them seriously. The skills taught in this module are to maximize the chances that a person's goals in a specific situation will be met, while at the same time not damaging (and, ideally, even enhancing) either interpersonal relationship or the person's self-respect.

The instructional content is divided into several segments. The first segment covers the basic interpersonal skills that are on the back of the diary cards and will be practiced for the rest of the treatment year. The se-

70

cond segment deals with identifying factors that contribute to interpersonal effectiveness, as well as things that interfere with being effective. The third segment addresses factors to consider before asking someone for something, saying no, or expressing an opinion. The module then moves into specific skills: self-cheerleading skills, skills for getting what one wants, for keeping the relationship, and skills for keeping one's self-respect.

This module is one of the most difficult to get through in just 8 weeks, and I have often added a week or two the first time I offer the module. It is especially easy to spend too much time on the first half, leaving too little time for teaching the actual behavioral skills (objectives, relationship, and self-respect effectiveness skills). At least half of the module should be devoted to these three sets of skills. This is essential, because a most important part of all interpersonal skills training programs is the in-session practice of new behaviors. Integrating behavioral practice of new behaviors within sessions, however, can be one of the most difficult parts for new therapists and for those not trained in behavior therapy. Thus, it can be very easy to just let it slip by in this module.

The beginning of the module includes a lot of more "cognitive" information and skills. These sections were put into the module because some of the topics actually do create difficulty for some borderline individuals, and I have conducted groups where members simply would not go on until we discussed one or more of these issues in depth. Thus, they are there if needed. The skills trainer may need to spend considerable time on some rather than others. Not all of these have to be covered in depth. Clients can read them between sessions, or they can be covered the next time the module is offered. If necessary for a particular client, the individual therapist can also give more attention to these segments, particularly setting goals and priorities and identifying factors that contribute to or interfere with being effective.

Content Outline

I. **Orient** clients to the skills to be learned in this module and the rationale for their importance.

A. Review Interpersonal Effectiveness Handout 1: Situations for Interpersonal Effectiveness.

Note to Leaders: This handout is intended to orient clients to times when the skills taught in this module might be very useful. Go over it briefly and move to the next handout. Spend more time on it, if necessary, later.

1. **Attending to relationships**
   a. Explain: "You need to attend to relationships to keep them in balance."
   b. Explain: "You need to attend to relationships to keep them from blowing up or otherwise ending."

Lecture Point: Relationships that are not attended to can create enormous stress. This stress then increases emotional vulnerability, and life can simply go downhill. Unattended relationships often blow up, and can end even when people want them to continue. The longer relationships remain unattended to, the harder they are to repair. The ability to repair relationships is much more important than keeping them from "tearing" in the first place.

2. **Balancing priorities vesus demands in life and relationships.**
   a. Explain: "Priorities are those things important to you, things that you want to do or get done."
   b. Explain: "Demands are those things other people want you to do, things other people want done."
   c. Explain: "Most troubles with priorities and demands are due to your own priorities' conflicting with other people's priorities. Thus, you need good interpersonal skills to maintain your own priorities and/or negotiate compromises."

Lecture Point: Balancing priorities and demands is the basic task for structuring one's life so that it is not too empty and not too full. Although this is difficult for everyone, it is especially difficult for the borderline individual, mainly because the ability to balance priorities and demands requires having requisite interpersonal capabilities and being able to use them in the appropriate situations.

Lecture Point: Describe what is meant by balancing priorities and demands in life. Generally, for the person who is overwhelmed, overcommitted, and doing too much, it means first sorting out what is more and less important and then saying no to some of the less important demands and priorities.

Discussion Point: Explain: "Importance, of course, is always relative. It is especially difficult to figure out when a particular demand is unimportant to you but important to others in your social network. However, if you overcommit yourself in order to maintain approval from another person, in the end the relationship itself will be harmed." Elicit feedback and discussion here to ferret out how much of a problem this is for participants.

Discussion Point: Just as a relationship may blow up if relationships are not attended to, at times an individual will blow up if priorities and demands in life are not attended to and balanced. Elicit examples.

Discussion Point: Some participants will report that the issue is not too many demands and priorities, but too few. This is especially likely if an individual is single, living alone, and not working. In these cases, the task is to create structure and increase demands rather than to decrease them. Interpersonal skills are likely to be needed here also. Elicit discussion and feedback.

Lecture Point: Draw a line on the blackboard. The left end of the line represents the beginning of a time period, and time moves along toward the right. Generally, if a person is overwhelmed, sooner or later she will either blow up or consider ending life. Often, this is when jobs are quit, suicide attempts are made, relationships are ended, and impulsive moves to other areas of the country occur.

Discussion Point: Elicit examples from participants of when they have become so overwhelmed that they have "blown up." Leaders: Share any examples from your own lives.

Lecture Point: The level of demands that can be easily tolerated varies over time and from person to person. To a certain extent, this level depends on a person's usual (or current) energy level, the amount of help and support forthcoming from the environment, and the person's emotional state of being. Thus, people are different, and these differences need not be judged.

Discussion Point: The borderline individual, like most persons, will often compare herself to other people and think that she should be able to do as much as these others. This comparison is often somewhat biased, and important factors are not taken into account. Also, borderline individuals, like others, often have a naive view of what other people can do, and therefore their beliefs about how much other people are doing are often overestimates. They set others on a pedestal and then feel inadequate when they cannot climb that same pedestal. What they fail to recognize is that the pedestal is often of their own creation; the other persons are in reality standing next to them. Elicit examples.

3. **Balancing the wants-to-shoulds ratio in life and relationships.**[1]

   a. Explain: "Wants include those things that you do because you want to do them, because they give you pleasure, or because you simply feel like doing them."

   b. Explain: "Shoulds are those things you do because you ought to do them or you have to do them for some reason."

Lecture Point: The essential idea here is that people often resort to impulsive and dysfunctional behaviors when the wants in their lives are out of balance with the shoulds. A healthy lifestyle requires some overall balance between wants and shoulds. A life that is dominated by wants often runs into trouble because responsibilities are not met and commitments are not kept. However, a life dominated by shoulds can lead to depression, frustration, and anger. Thus, a balance in the long run is essential. These points need to be discussed in detail, since in my experience borderline clients often have trouble understanding the concept here.

Lecture Point: Draw on the board a balancing scale to give a visual representation of what you are talking about. Although people can sometimes balance the wants-to-shoulds ratio without using any interpersonal skills, most of the time interpersonal skills are necessary. At times it requires getting one's opinions taken seriously, getting other people to do things, or saying no to unwanted requests.

Discussion Point: Query participants about the current balance in their lives and what they think is needed to get their lives back in balance. It is essential here, besides getting the concept across, to relate balancing the wants-to-shoulds ratio to using interpersonal skills. Elicit from participants examples of how other people are critical to their keeping the wants-to-shoulds ratio in balance.

4. **Building mastery and self-respect.**

   a. Explain: "You build mastery when you do things that make you feel competent and effective."

   b. Explain: "You build self-respect when you stand up for yourself, express your own beliefs and opinions, follow your wise mind, and do what you believe is right and moral."

Lecture Point: Mastery is the opposite of active passivity. (See Chapter 3 of the text for a description of active passivity.) Building mastery requires doing things that are difficult, that involve a challenge. Hopelessness is the enemy of mastery. Overcoming obstacles is one route to mastery. Most successful people in this world do not have fewer obstacles; they just get up after falling down more often than unsuccessful people do. Getting up after falling down is mastery. Falling down is irrelevant. The drive to mastery seems to be innate. Small children learning how to walk they keep falling down and getting up, falling down and getting up.

Discussion Point: Discuss with participants what has happened to their ability to get up after falling down, their sense of mastery. Obviously, if a person never succeeds at a task, the sense of mastery won't grow. Children do not try to walk before they crawl. They do not try to do things they simply cannot do. If they try, they soon cease and try something else they can do.

Discussion Point: Explain: "If you are raised in a punishing family, one that invalidates difficulties, then it is difficult to achieve a sense of mastery." Most borderline individuals have difficulty achieving a sense of mastery. They compare themselves to others and fall short. It is like a person with no legs comparing herself to runners with two legs; the comparison is faulty. However, in the case of legs, the handicap is obvious. In the case of emotional difficulties, the handicaps are less obvious. Get feedback.

Lecture Point: Often the most difficult situations to master are interpersonal. If people are shy, they do not want to go places. They find it hard to ask for what they need, hard to say no, hard to express their opinions firmly, and hard to attend to relationships. Practicing interpersonal skills builds mastery.

Discussion Point: Elicit from participants times when they have done things that reduce their own sense of mastery. When have they enhanced their sense of mastery? How would they like to improve?

   B. Present **two types of interpersonal skills to be taught:**

      1. Asking for things, making requests, initiating discussions.

      2. Saying no, resisting pressure, maintaining a position or point of view.

Discussion Point: Discuss with participants how they view their own interpersonal skills. Some individuals will be good at asking for things but terrible at saying no, whereas others can say no but cannot ask for anything. Still others are deficient across the board. Make it clear that sometimes individuals have appropriate skills in some situational contexts but not in others. For example, some people may be quite adequate at saying no to strangers but not to friends; others may be able to ask for help from friends but not from their bosses. Elicit from each person the types of skills she feels she has and the situations she is good in, as well as areas that need further work. Leaders: Feel free here to share with participants your own areas of strength and weakness. The major goal here is for clients to see the relevance of interpersonal skills training to their own lives by seeing areas in which they need improvement. Also, the discussion serves to normalize the notion of skill deficits by highlighting that everyone has areas in which she can improve her skills.

In my experience, some borderline clients are exceptionally skilled in many interpersonal situations and may present as if they do not need interpersonal skills training. However, a closer discussion, especially of var-ious situational contexts, will reveal that almost everyone can use some skills training. Therefore, even with a very skilled person, make every effort to identify areas where that person can use improvement.

> **II. Review Interpersonal Effectiveness Handout 2: Goals of Interpersonal Effectiveness.**

> **Note to Leaders:** Homework practice sheet for these skills is Interpersonal Effectiveness Homework Sheet 1: Goals and Priorities in Interpersonal Situations.

   A. **Objectives effectiveness.** Explain: "Objectives effectiveness refers to attaining your objectives or goals in a situation. The idea with these skills is to get what you want in an interaction, for your wishes to be taken seriously. They include the following:

      1. Standing up for your rights in such a way that they are taken seriously.

      2. Requesting others to do something in such a way that they do it.

      3. Refusing unwanted or unreasonable requests and making the refusal stick.

      4. Resolving interpersonal conflict.

      5. Getting your opinion or point of view taken seriously."

Lecture Point: Borderline individuals often believe that all failures to get what they want from someone else are failures in skills. They have difficulty seeing that sometimes the environment is simply impervious to even the most skilled individuals. Thus, when they fail to get what they want using interpersonal skills, they may either fall back into hopelessness, try an aggressive response, or threaten (i.e., blackmail) other people if they don't give them what they want. Thus, although increased interpersonal skills should increase the probability of getting objectives met, they are not a guarantee. Distress tolerance and reality acceptance are indispensable parts of interpersonal skills.

Discussion Point: Get feedback. When have participants used really good skills but not gotten what they wanted? How did they feel afterwards?

   B. **Relationship effectiveness:** Explain: "Relationship effectiveness is the art of maintaining or even improving an interpersonal relationship while you try to get what you want—that is, while you try to obtain your objectives. At its best, you will get what you want, and the person may like or respect you even more than before. These skills are as follows:

1. Acting in a way that makes the other person actually want to give you what you are asking for or feel good about your saying no.
2. Balancing immediate goals with the good of the long-term relationship."

Lecture Point: Explain: "If the main goal of the interaction is to get the other person to approve of you more, stop criticizing or rejecting you, stay with you, or the like, then enhancing the relationship is the objective and should be considered under objectives effectiveness. In that case, relationship effectiveness refers to choosing a way to go about improving or keeping the relationship that does not at the same time damage the relationship over the long run."

Discussion Point: Elicit from participants times they have risked a long term relationship for a short-term relationship gain. Examples may include attempting or threatening suicide to keep someone from leaving, or attacking another person for voicing criticism.

Lecture Point: Borderline individuals, of course, are highly concerned with maintaining relationships, approval, and liking. They are often willing to sacrifice personal goals for the sake of interpersonal relationships. Frequently, they operate under the myth that if they sacrifice their own needs and wants to other people, their relationships will go more smoothly, approval will be ever forthcoming, and no problems will arise. The key problem with this approach to life is that it doesn't work; it is ineffective. Make this point especially clear.

Lecture Point: Draw a time line on the blackboard, as before. At the left end of the time line mark the beginning of a relationship. Then move the chalk toward the right as if time were marching on and discuss how a relationship goes if a person constantly subverts her own needs for the sake of a relationship. Although for some time a person can survive in such a relationship, at some point in time the frustrations that build up will have to be dealt with—usually at the point where frustrations are long-standing, the needs that have been unmet are large, and the sense of inequity is extreme. One of two things will happen. The frustrated individual will (1) blow up and thereby risk losing the relationship through the other person's rejecting her and walking out, or (2) in frustration leave the relationship herself. Either way, the relationship comes to an end or is in serious jeopardy.

Discussion Point: Engage the participants in a discussion of how this pattern has worked in their lives. Usually someone can give examples of how she has blown up. Indeed, for borderline individuals, parasuicide is often a method of getting someone to take your feelings and opinions seriously or of getting other people to change their behavior. It is a good example of the kind of behavior that shows up at the right-hand end of the continuum. Other dysfunctional behaviors can also be used as examples. It is important to elicit from participants how blowing up or walking out of relationships inadvertently jeopardizes their own goals. Clients may have great difficulty seeing this point. In my experience, borderline individuals often believe that these extreme behaviors not only are effective but are the only behaviors possible given the circumstances of their lives. It is essential at this point to develop some insight into how these strategies are self-defeating in the long run.

Discussion Point: A key idea is that by not using interpersonal skills earlier in the sequence, the person has in fact jeopardized a relationship's very existence instead of keeping it together. The idea here, of course, is to try to highlight how employing interpersonal skills will not only enhance relationships but improve a person's chances of obtaining interpersonal and social approval rather than the opposite. A strategy that is sometimes useful at this point and at many other points is to ask participants to imagine another person's engaging in extreme interpersonal behaviors with them, such as parasuicide or blowing up. How would it feel? From that perspective, individuals often find it easier to see the dysfunctional nature of the behaviors. The main goal here is to elicit clients' commitment to the value of learning and practicing interpersonal skills. Of course, such a commitment is likely to vanish in the actual situation where employing the skills is necessary; nonetheless, obtaining it is the first step in the process of shaping interpersonal skills.

C. **Self-respect effectiveness.** Explain: "Self-respect effectiveness is maintaining or improving your good feelings about yourself, and respecting your own values and beliefs, while you try to attain your objectives. It includes the following:

1. Acting in ways that fit your sense of morality.
2. Acting in ways that make you feel competent."

Lecture Point: Giving in for the sake of approval, lying to please others, and the like all diminishes self-respect over time. Acting helpless also diminishes self-respect in the long term. Even if acting helpless is strategic—that is, deliberately calculated to get someone to do something—if overused the strategy will inevitably lead to reduced mastery. This point is very important. Acting helpless on purpose, when it works, can give a temporary sense of mastery. It is the overuse of this approach that causes problems.

Discussion Point: Elicit from participants times when they have done things that reduce their own sense of self-respect. When have they enhanced their sense of self-respect? Where do they need to improve their skills?

III. **Explain the relationship** among the three types of effectiveness.

A. All three types of effectiveness enter into and must be considered in every conflict or interpersonal problem situation.

B. One or more types of effectiveness may be more or less important in a given situation.

C. How effective a behavior is in a particular situation depends on a person's priorities.

IV. **Give examples** of situations and goals.

A. Landlord keeps deposit unfairly (**objective** most important).

1. Objective: Getting deposit back.
2. Relationship: Keeping landlord's good will and liking, or at least keeping good reference.
3. Self-respect: Not losing self-respect by getting too emotional, "fighting dirty," giving in.

B. Best friend wants to come over and discuss a problem; person wants to go to bed (**relationship** most important).

1. Objective: Going to bed.
2. Relationship: Keeping good relationship with friend.
3. Self-respect: Balancing caring for friend with caring for self.

C. Person wants a raise; her boss wants sex in return (**self-respect** most important).

1. Objective: Getting raise; staying out of bed with boss.
2. Relationship: Keeping boss's respect and good will.
3. Self-respect: Not violating own moral code.

Discussion Point: Have participants generate other situations and identify the objective(s) in the situation, the relationship issue, and the self-respect issue. Discuss priorities for each situation. Continue generating situations until it is clear that the participants have grasped the essential points.

V. Review Interpersonal Effectiveness Handout 3: Factors Reducing Interpersonal Effectiveness.

Note to Leaders: Homework practice sheet for these and following skills is Interpersonal Effectiveness Homework Sheet 2: Observing and Describing Interpersonal Situations.

A. **Skill deficits.** Explain: "When you have skill deficits, you actually don't know what to say or how to act. You don't know how you should behave to obtain your objectives."

Lecture Point: Describe the role of lack of ability to behave in a certain way; this is very different from motivational explanations of behavior. Emphasize that people learn social behaviors by observing someone else do them first, practicing them, and refining them until they can be used to obtain good results. People sometimes don't have enough opportunities to observe; therefore, they don't learn the behaviors. Or they don't have the chance to practice the behaviors they do observe. Describe how a person can have skills in one set of situations but not in another, or in one mood but not in another, or in one frame of mind but not in another.

Discussion Point: Elicit examples of having variable skills, depending on the situation or mood.

B. **Worry thoughts.** Explain: "Worry thoughts may get in the way of your ability to behave. You have the capability, but it is interfered with by your worry thoughts."

1. Worrying about bad consequences (e.g., "They won't like me," "She will think I am stupid").
2. Worrying about whether one deserves to get what one wants (e.g., "I am such a bad person I don't deserve this").
3. Worrying about not being effective and calling oneself names (e.g., "I won't do it right," "I'll probably fall apart," "I'm so stupid").

C. **Emotional reactions.** Explain: "Emotions may get in the way of our ability to behave. You have the capability, but it is interfered with by your emotions. You may get angry or anxious, or feel frustrated and guilty, because of how you think about situations or because you don't know what to do. Emotions can keep you from acting or emotions can be so strong that emotional actions, words, and face and body expressions are automatic, overwhelming skills."

Lecture Point: Emotional reactions can be automatic reactions to situations, based on previous conditioning. Or they can be a result of believing the myths to be discussed below (or other myths).

D. **Indecision.** Explain: "You may not be able to decide what to do. You have the capability, but it is interfered with by your indecision."

1. Ambivalence about priorities.
2. Inability to decide how to balance asking (saying no) with not asking (saying yes).

Discussion Point: Discuss tendency to go to extremes of asking (saying no) versus not asking (giving in). Also discuss tendency to go to extremes of belief: complete neediness (and asking in a clinging, begging, grasping or hysterical manner) versus complete self-sufficiency (and never asking, saying yes to everything), or, complete worthiness (and asking in an inappropriately demanding manner or refusing belligerently) versus complete unworthiness (and never asking or saying no). Elicit examples.

    E. **Environment.** Explain: "Environmental factors may preclude effectiveness. At times even the most skilled individuals cannot be effective at getting what they want, keeping others liking them, or behaving in ways that they respect."

      1. When the environment is powerful, other people may simply refuse to give a person what she wants, or they may have the authority to make her do what they want her to do. Saying no or insisting on rights may have very negative consequences.

      2. Sometimes there simply is no way for a person to get what she wants or to say no and keep the other person liking her. People may be threatened, jealous, or envious, or have any number of other reasons for not liking someone.

      3. When a person is faced with a conflict, and achieving an objective is very important (e.g., food for her children, medical care when she is sick), she may have to act in ways that damage her pride or otherwise hurt her self-respect.

Note to Leaders: Borderline individuals seem to have a very unrealistic view of the world and of what skilled people can do. In particular, they seem to believe that if they just ask correctly or are skilled enough, they can get whatever they want or need. The idea that people often don't get what they want or need isn't clear to them. Thus, they almost always blame themselves if they are ineffective at getting what they want. This self-blame then often generates anger and frustration. The belief that people can always get what they want and need precludes the necessity of developing distress tolerance skills. Without such skills, frustration often turns into anger. Be very careful on this point, especially during homework discussions.

    F. **Interplay of factors.** Explain: "The less you know, the more you worry, the worse you feel, the more you can't decide what to do, the more ineffective you are, the more you worry, and so on. Or the more you experience nongiving and authoritarian environments, the more you worry, the less you practice, the less you know, the worse you feel, the more you can't decide what to do, and so on."

┌───┐
│ **VI. Review Interpersonal Effectiveness Hand-** │
│ **out 4: Myths about Interpersonal** │
│ **Effectiveness.** │
└───┘

Lecture Point: All people have some worries about standing up for themselves, expressing opinions, saying no, and so on. Sometimes worries are based on myths about interpersonal behavior. One way to counteract these worries and myths is to try to argue against them logically. Another way is to experiment in the world and see whether they are really true. Counteracting worry thoughts and myths is an example of cognitive modification or cognitive therapy. It can sometimes be useful in getting people to do things they really want to do but are afraid to do. Challenges to myths can be used to challenge worries that crop up about trying interpersonal skills.

Discussion Point: Use the devil's advocate technique to discuss myths about interpersonal effectiveness. The task of participants is to develop challenges or counter arguments against the myths. These challenges can be used as cheerleading statements later to help clients get themselves to act effectively. Everyone write challenges down as participants think them up.

Note to Leaders: In the devil's advocate strategy, you present myths and then argue in favor of them, giving rather extreme positive statements, and thus getting participants to argue the case for the counterstatements. The discussion on each statement should be resolved by transcending the extremes to find a synthesis or balancing point of view. Not every myth has to be discussed in the session; the participants should be included in choosing which ones to go over in the session. (See Chapter 7 of the text for further discussion of this strategy.) A homework assignment might be to have clients complete the challenges not done during the session. Another assignment might be to observe themselves over the week and write down any other myths that they operate by. They should also think up challenges.

Discussion Point: There are a number of ways to discuss these myths. One way is to read out each myth and have participants circle the myth if they agree with it. Generally, you first have to have a discussion about the difference between intellectual agreement and emotional agreement. You can also add "wise mind" agreement. Explain: "Intellectual agreement is thinking that something is true; your rational mind tells you so. However, you may feel it is not true or know it is not. Emotional agreement is feeling that something is true, or reacting emotionally as if it is true. In these cases, you may believe and/or know that it is not. In wise mind, you know in your heart of hearts that something is or is not true." After the participants have marked myths as true or not, read the myths again and ask who agrees with each myth, who circled it as true. Others who did not circle the myth should be encouraged to offer challenges.

VII. Review Interpersonal Effectiveness Handout 5: Cheerleading Statements for Interpersonal Effectiveness.

A. **Cheerleading statements** are statements that people make to themselves (i.e., self-statements) in order to give themselves permission to ask for what they need or want, to say no, and to act effectively. There are several types:

1. Statements that provide the courage to act effectively.

2. Statements that help in preparing for the situation—in getting ready to be effective, to focus on what works.

3. Statements that counteract myths about interpersonal behavior—unrealistic beliefs and assumptions that interfere with being effective.

Lecture Point: Remind participants that some of the challenges they have generated to myths about interpersonal effectiveness can also be used as cheerleading statements. Encourage participants to select cheerleading statements that are well suited to them—that counteract their own myths and unrealistic beliefs.

Note to Leaders: As with any new skill, it is essential that clients practice the new skill. For cheerleading statements, they can do this in two ways—imaginarily or by thinking out loud.

B. **Imaginal practice.**

1. Instruct participants to close their eyes and imagine the situation you will be describing. Instruct them to imagine that they are in the situation, not observing the situation from the outside.

2. Describe an interpersonal conflict situation (see Handout 7 for list of practice situations, or use situations developed by clients). Give participants enough time to imagine themselves in the scene. (The first few times, check on how well participants are getting into the scenes, in order to gauge how to describe the situation.)

3. While participants are imagining themselves in the situation, instruct them to imagine themselves saying a cheerleading statement to themselves: "Say it in imagination as if you mean it."

4. Share with all participants cheerleading statements each person uses.

C. **Thinking-out-loud practice.**

1. As above, describe a situation. You can have participants close their eyes and imagine being in the situation, as above, or not.

2. Go around the room rapidly and ask each participant to say a cheerleading statement out loud. (More than one person can use the same statement.)

3. You can use any of the procedures described below for role playing for thinking-out-loud practice.

Discussion Point: Use the devil's advocate strategy to go over some of the cheerleading statements, especially if new ones are generated.

VIII. Review Interpersonal Effectiveness Handout 6: Options for Intensity of Asking or Saying No, and Factors to Consider in Deciding.

Lecture Point: Being interpersonally effective requires thinking through whether it is appropriate to ask for something or to say no to a request. For example, a person who is sick might ask her healthy roommate to bring her a glass of orange juice. When the person asking is healthy and the roommate is sick, it would clearly be inappropriate to do so. The answer is not usually so black and white, however, contrary to what the average borderline individual thinks. Instead, there are levels of asking and levels of saying no.

A. **Options for intensity of asking and saying no.** Explain:

6. **Asking:** Ask firmly, insist. **Saying no:** Refuse firmly, don't give in.

5. **Asking:** Ask firmly, resist no. **Saying no:** Refuse firmly, resist giving in.

4. **Asking:** Ask firmly, take no. **Saying no:** Refuse firmly, but reconsider.

3. **Asking:** Ask tentatively, take no. **Saying no:** Express unwillingness.

2. **Asking:** Hint openly, take no. **Saying no:** Express unwillingness, but say yes.

1. **Asking:** Hint indirectly, take no. **Saying no:** Express hesitancy, say yes.

0. **Asking:** Don't ask, don't hint. **Saying no:** Do what other wants without being asked.

B. **Factors to consider in deciding on intensity of response.**

1. **Priorities: Objectives?** If objectives are very important, the intensity of the response should to be higher.

Relationship? Often, relationship issues are such that one is willing to trade an objective for keeping the other person happy. If so, the intensity of the response should be lower.

Self-Respect? Self-respect issues may lead to a more or a less intense response, depending on how one feels about the outcome and the behavior.

2. **Capability:** If the other person has what one wants, the intensity of asking should be higher.

If one does **not** have (and, therefore cannot give or do) what the other person wants, the intensity of saying no should be higher.[2]

3. **Timelessness:** If this is a good time to ask (other person is "in the mood" for listening and paying attention; he or she is likely to say yes to a request) the intensity of asking should be higher.

If this is **not** a bad time for one to say no, the intensity of saying no should be higher.

4. **Homework:** If one knows all the facts necessary to support a request, and both the goal and the request are clear, intensity of asking should be higher.

If the other person's request is **not** clear, the intensity of saying no should be higher.

5. **Authority:** If one is responsible for directing the other person or telling him or her what to do, the intensity of asking should be higher.

If the other person does **not** have authority or what the person is asking is **not** within his or her authority, the intensity of saying no should be higher.

6. **Rights:** If the other person is required by law or moral code to give what one wants, the intensity of asking should be higher.

If one is **not** required to give what the other person wants (saying no would **not** violate the other person's rights), the intensity of saying no should be higher.

7. **Relationship:** If what one wants is appropriate to the current relationship, the intensity of asking should be higher.

If what the other person wants is **not** appropriate to the current relationship, the intensity of saying no should be higher.

8. **Reciprocity:** If one has done at least as much for the other person as one is requesting, and is willing to give if the other

person says yes, the intensity of asking should be higher.

If one does **not** owe the other person a favor, or the other person does **not** usually reciprocate, the intensity of saying no should be higher.

9. **Long versus short term:** If being submissive will result in peace now but create problems in the long run, the intensity of asking should be higher.

If giving in and getting short-term peace now is **not** more important than the long-term welfare of the relationship, the intensity of saying no should be higher.[2]

10. **Respect:** If one usually does things for oneself and is careful to avoid acting helpless when this is not the case, the intensity of asking should be higher.

If saying no will **not** result in bad feelings about oneself, and if wise mind says no, the intensity of saying no should be higher.

C. Homework sheets can be used in deciding whether to ask for something or say no to a request.

1. On the left side, participants should count the number of "Yes" responses. If there are more "Yes" than "No" responses, then participants should make the request. The more "Yes" responses, the more intense the request should be.

2. On the right side, participants should count up the number of "No" responses. If there are more "No" than "Yes" responses, then participants should say no to a request made of them. The more "No" responses, the more intense saying no to the other person should be.

IX. **Prepare to present skills** for interpersonal effectiveness.

A. Note that skills will be learned for enhancing each type of effectiveness (**objectives, relationship, self-respect**).

Note to Leaders: The skills are designed for effectiveness and do not necessarily follow rules clients may have learned in assertiveness classes. There are probably many other skills that would be just as effective. Clients should be encouraged to suggest other skills they have found effective.

Note to Leaders: An essential component of interpersonal skills training is behavioral rehearsal, both in sessions and between sessions as homework. With the exception of the first session, some time must be set aside each session for behavioral rehearsal. You must convey a sense of expectation and encouragement that everyone will participate in role playing.

  B. Stress necessity of **behavioral rehearsal** (role-playing) in sessions to learn new skills.

  C. Stress necessity of **homework practice** in learning to use new skills where needed.

> **Give out Interpersonal Effectiveness Handout 7: Suggestions for Interpersonal Effectiveness Practice.**

---

  1. Emphasize: "If a situation arises between sessions where you can ask for something or say no, do it and try to use your skills."
  2. Explain: "If nothing arises in daily life to give you the opportunity to practice, you need to dream up situations where you can practice. That is, do not just wait for a situation to arise where you can practice. Actively search out situations."
  3. This list has lots of ideas for practice, or participants can make up their own situations.

Discussion Point: Get feedback. Discuss objections to doing things on the list. Be flexible here. Borderline clients may be unable to do many of the things on the list. Remember your principles of shaping here. (See Chapter 10 of text.)

> **X. Review Interpersonal Effectiveness Handout 8: Guidelines for Objectives Effectiveness: Getting What You Want.**

> **Note to Leaders:** Homework practice sheet for these and following skills is Interpersonal Effectiveness Homework Sheet 3: Using Interpersonal Effectiveness Skills.

  A. Review definition of objective effectiveness.
  B. A way to remember the skills for objective effectiveness is to remember the term **"DEAR MAN"**:[3]

> **D**escribe
> **E**xpress
> **A**ssert
> **R**einforce
>
> (stay) **M**indfully
> **A**ppear confident
> **N**egotiate

  1. **Describe the situation.** Explain: "When necessary, briefly describe the situation you are reacting to. Stick to the facts. **No judgmental statements.** Be objective." Give examples: "I've been working here for 2 years and have not gotten a raise, even though my performance reviews have been very positive." "This is the third time you've asked this week for a ride home from work."
  2. **Express feelings or opinions about the situation clearly.** Explain: "Describe how you feel or what you believe about the situation. Don't expect the other person to read your mind or know how you feel. For instance, give a brief rationale for a request or for saying no." Give examples: "I believe that I deserve a raise." "I'm getting home so late that it is really hard for me and my family. But I also really enjoy giving you rides home, and it is hard to say no."

Lecture Point: These two skills are not always necessary. For example, a person might simply ask a family member going to the grocery store to get some orange juice (without saying "We're out and I'd like some"). In a hot, stuffy room, the person could ask someone else to open a window (without necessarily saying, "the room is stuffy and I'm feeling hot"). In saying no to a request, the person might simply say, "No, I can't do it." Every participant, however, should learn and practice each of the skills.

  3. **Assert wishes.** Explain: "Ask for what you want. Say no clearly. Don't expect people to know what you want them to do if you don't tell them. Ask them for what you *want*. Don't tell them what they *should* do. Don't beat around the bush, never really asking or saying no." Give examples: "I would like a raise. Can you give it to me?" "But I have to say no tonight. I can't give you a ride home so often."

Lecture Point: These skills have to do mostly with being clear, concise, and assertive. The idea is to avoid beating around the bush or expecting others to be mind readers. The point to be conveyed is that a person just has to bite the bullet and ask or say no.

  4. **Reinforce.** Explain: "Remember to reward people who respond positively to you when you ask for something, say no, or express an opinion. Sometimes it is effective to reinforce people before they respond to you positively by telling them the positive effects of getting what you want or need." Give ex-

amples: "I will be a lot happier and probably more productive if I get a salary that reflects my value to the company." "Thanks for being so understanding, I really appreciate it."

Discussion Point: The basic idea here is that if other people do not gain from complying with a request, or taking no for an answer, at least some of the time they may stop responding in a positive way. The notion of behaviors being controlled by consequences instead of by concepts of "good" and "bad" or "right" and "wrong" can be particularly difficult for some clients to grasp. Discuss this idea with participants.

Practice Exercise: Once a chunk of material is presented and discussed, move to rehearsal, where the material just learned can be practiced. Techniques are as follows:

1. Rapid rehearsal can be accomplished by going about the room and having each person briefly rehearse a particular skill immediately after it is presented or discussed. For example, participants can be asked to describe situations, express feelings or opinions about the situation, ask for something or refuse directly, or make a reinforcing comment. You can have everyone practice on the same situation (which either you or the participants can make up) or have each person use a situation from her own life. Practicing on the same situation is usually quicker if time is of the essence. Use this procedure at least once after presenting each individual skill.

2. Participants can role-play a situation, taking turns playing the person who is asking or saying no and the other person in the situation. Taking the part of the other person can be very important to give clients an idea of what it feels like when someone else uses behavioral skills on them.

3. One person can rehearse (role-play) a situation with you, the leader during the session. Usually, this is done when the participant is describing homework and it seems useful for her to try acting differently in the situation right away. It can also be used when a participant wants (or needs) help with particular types of situations.

4. If a client simply cannot role-play or refuses to do so, present the situation in story fashion: Ask, "Then what would you say?"; wait for a response; and then say, "OK, then the other person says . . . What would you say next?"

5. If the client refuses even this sort of dialogue, then ask her to role-play the situation in her head and imagine giving a skilled response. Do a fair amount of prompting to guide the client's attention and focus.

Note to Leaders: Role playing is often the most difficult procedure for therapists with little experience in behavior therapy; nonetheless, it is essential. (You might try the role-play procedures with a friend to get some practice.) **Do not sacrifice rehearsal in order to present more material.** Role playing can also be hard for clients at first, but with experience it gets easier. At the beginning, you sometimes have to pull or drag them through the practice. The most important thing with a reluctant role player is that you not fall out of role, even if she does. Just keep responding to her as if you are actually in the role-play situation. Usually, this will do the trick and the person will get back into the role play.

5. **(stay) Mindful.** Explain: "Keep your focus on your objectives in the situation. Maintain your position and don't be distracted onto another topic. There are two useful techniques here."

a. **"Broken record."** Explain: "Keep asking, saying no, or expressing your opinion over and over and over."

Lecture Point: This is perhaps one of the most important skills taught during this segment. It is also one of the skills clients can learn most readily, as it is easy to do and remember. The idea to get across is that a person doesn't have to think up something different to say each time; she can keep saying exactly the same thing. The key here is to keep a "mellow" voice tone—"kill them with sweetness," so to speak. The strength is in the persistence of maintaining the position. Go around and practice this with each person.

b. **Ignore.** Explain: "If another person attacks, threatens, or tries to change the subject, ignore their threats, comments, or attempts to divert you. Just keep making your point."

Discussion Point: The key idea to get across here is that if a person pays attention to attacks, responds to them in any way, or lets them divert her in the slightest, then she is giving the other person control of the interaction. If the person wants to respond to the attacks, that is another issue and can be dealt with in another discussion, or after this one is finished. Once clients get the hang of this skill, it can be quite fun to use. Get feedback on this point from participants, paying special attention to their beliefs that they have to respond to every criticism or attack made by another.

Note to Leaders: This skill, combined with the "broken record," makes for a very effective strategy in maintaining a refusal or putting pressure on someone to comply with a request. When the other person attacks, one should simply replay the "broken record." It is extremely difficult to keep attacking or criticizing a person who doesn't respond or "play the game." But, it is a lot harder than it looks. The only way for clients to get the hang of this skill is to practice. **Be sure to practice both of these skills with all participants.** Also, it can be a nice idea to have participants practice with each other, to see what having their own attacks and diversion strategies ignored or having another person keep repeating a request, opinion, or refusal feels like. The key to the "broken record" and ignoring attacks is to keep hostility out of one's voice, but keep on track.

   6. **Appear confident.** Explain: "Use a confident voice tone and display a confident physical manner with appropriate eye contact. Such a manner conveys to both the other person and yourself that you are efficacious and deserve respect for what you want. No stammering, whispering, staring at the floor, retreating, saying you're not sure, or the like."

Discussion Point: How confident to act in a given situation is a judgment call. A person needs to talk a fine line between appearing arrogant and appearing too apologetic. Elicit examples from participants.

   7. **Negotiate.** Explain: "Be willing to give to get. Offer and ask for alternative solutions to the problem. Reduce your request. Maintain your no, but offer to do something else or solve the problem another way. An alternative technique is to turn the tables."

      a. **Turn the table.** Explain: "Turn the problem over to the other person. Ask for alternative solutions." Give examples: "What do you think we should do?" "I'm not able to say yes, and you really seem to want me to. What can we do here?" "How can we solve this problem?"

Discussion Point: Negotiating or turning the tables is useful when ordinary requesting or refusing is getting nowhere. There are many variations on the negotiating strategy. Get participants to discuss any time they have used it.

   C. Use objectives effectiveness in really difficult situations.

      1. Explain: "Sometimes other people have really good skills themselves, and keep refusing your legitimate requests or pestering you to do something you don't want to do."

      2. In such cases, the same **"DEAR MAN"** skills should be used, except that the focus should be changed to the current in-teraction with the person (the person's behavior right now). In particular, the "DEAR" skills change as follows:

      a. **Describe the current interaction.** Explain: "If the 'broken record' and ignoring don't work, make a statement about what is happening between you and the person now, but without imputing motives." Give examples: "You keep asking me over and over, even though I have already said no," *not* "You just don't want to hear what I am saying."

      b. **Express feelings or opinions about the interaction.** Explain: "For instance, in the middle of an interaction that is not going well, you can express your feelings of discomfort in the situation." Give examples: "I'm not sure you understand what I am asking," or "I'm starting to feel angry about this."

      c. **Assert wishes in the situation.** Explain: "For example, when a person is refusing a request, suggest that you put the conversation off until another time. Give the other person a chance to think about it. When another person is pestering you, ask him or her to stop it."

      d. **Reinforce.** Explain: "When saying no to someone who keeps asking, or when someone won't take your opinion seriously, suggest ending the conversation since you aren't going to change your mind anyway."

XI. Review Interpersonal Effectiveness Handout 9: Guidelines for Relationship Effectiveness: Keeping the Relationship.

   A. Review definition of relationship effectiveness.
   B. A way to remember the skills for relationship effectiveness is to remember the word **"GIVE"** **(DEAR MAN, GIVE):**

   (be) **G**entle
   (act) **I**nterested
   Validate
   (use an) **E**asy manner

   1. (be) **G**entle. Explain: "Be courteous and temperate in your approach. People tend to respond to gentleness more than they do to harshness. In particular, avoid attacks, threats, and judgments."

      a. **No attacks.** Explain: "This is really pretty clear. People won't like you if you threaten them, attack them, or express much anger directly."

b. **No threats.** Explain: "Don't make 'manipulative' statements or hidden threats. Don't say, 'I'll kill myself if you . . .' Tolerate a no to requests. Stay in the discussion even if it gets painful. Exit gracefully."

Note to Leaders: This point may be very sensitive with some clients. I usually present it as if it is not sensitive and ask whether anyone has a problem with making threats. The idea is to normalize the interpersonal behavior (making threats "manipulating") that they have been accused of by others. Acknowledge how hard it is to stop such behavior.

Discussion Point: Usually the question will come up of how a person can communicate suicidal ideation in such a way that it is not a threat and that others do not take it as a threat. This is a good question. Generally, the best way is for the person to couple the communication with a statement that she wants to work on her urges to harm or kill herself. Explain: "The idea is to make it sound as if you are taking responsibility for not harming or killing yourself rather than making it the other person's responsibility. When others feel like that (even if you did not cause it), they usually say that you are threatening or manipulating them. In general, if you say that you feel like you are going to kill or harm yourself, but at the same time say that you want help or that you know you can control yourself, it is not a threat. Saying that you are going to commit suicide or harm yourself if someone else doesn't come through for you, do what you want, cure you, or make things better —or even implying this—is a threat."

c. **No judging.** Explain: "No name calling, 'shoulds,' or implied put downs in voice or manner. No guilt trips."

Discussion Point: This point is woven throughout all of the skills. But, it is so important that it is emphasized as a separate skill. Elicit from participants times when they have felt judged by others. Try a role-play to see what it feels like to be judged.

2. **(act) Interested.** Explain: "Be interested in the other person. Listen to the other person's point of view, opinion, reasons for saying no, or reasons for making a request of you. Don't interrupt, try to talk it over, or the like. Be sensitive to the other person's desire to have the discussion at a later time, if that's what the person wants. Be patient."

Lecture Point: Explain: "People feel better about you if you are interested in them and if you give them time and space to respond to you."

3. **Validate.** Explain: "Validate or acknowledge the other person's feelings, wants, difficulties, and opinions about the situation. Be nonjudgmental out loud."

Lecture Point: Explain: "Validating often requires you to read the other person's mind. Figure out what problems the person might be having with your request or your saying no. Then acknowledge those feelings or problems." Give examples: "I know that you are very busy, but . . . ." "I can see that this is really important to you, ..." "I know this will take you out of your way a bit, ..."

Note to Leaders: Clients can practice validating others even if a conflict situation does not arise—that is, they don't make a request or say no. Validating is simply a good, all-purpose skill. More than any other skill, this one has the potential to affect the quality of relationships.

4. **(use an) Easy manner.** Explain: "Try to be lighthearted. Use a little humor. Smile. Ease the other person along. Wheedle. Soothe. This is the difference between the 'soft sell' and the 'hard sell.' Be political."

Lecture Point: People don't like to be bullied, pushed, or made to feel guilty. Although people often say that borderline individuals are manipulators, a *really* good manipulator makes other people like giving in. The premise in DBT is that borderline individuals need to learn to be better at manipulating—inducing others to do what they want them to do.

C. Use relationship effectiveness in important relationships.

1. Explain: "Sometimes you have to sacrifice the short-term relationship for a few hours or days for the sake of the long-term relationship. You have to stand up for yourself and allow the other person to be angry, sad, or disappointed."

2. In important relationships, the **"DEAR MAN"** skills are also relationship effectiveness skills. Explain: "When you use 'DEAR MAN' appropriately, you take the burden off the other person of always having to take care of you."

XI. Review Interpersonal Effectiveness Handout 10: Guidelines for Self-Respect Effectiveness: Keeping Your Respect for Yourself.

A. Review definition of self-respect effectiveness.

B. A way to remember the skills for self-respect

effectiveness is to remember the word **"FAST"** (DEAR MAN, GIVE FAST):

> (be) **F**air
> (no) **A**pologies
> **S**tick to values
> (be) **T**ruthful

1. **(be) F̲air:** Explain: "Be fair to yourself and the other person in your attempts to solve the problem."

Lecture Point: Explain: "It is hard to like yourself over the long haul if you consistently take advantage of other people. You may get what you want, but at the risk of your ability to respect yourself."

2. **(no) A̲pologies.** Explain: "When apologies are warranted, of course they are appropriate. But don't engage in overapologetic behavior. No apologizing for being alive, for making a request at all. No apologies for having an opinion, for disagreeing. Apologies imply that you are wrong—that you are the one making a mistake. This can reduce your sense of self-efficacy over time."

Lecture Point: Like telling a lie, making apologies can at times enhance relationship effectiveness. The need to enhance the relationship must be balanced with the need to enhance self-respect. Excessive apologies, however, often get on other people's nerves and usually reduce both relationship and self-respect effectiveness.

3. **S̲tick to values.** Explain: "Don't sell out your values or integrity just to get your objective or keep a person liking you. Be clear on what, in your opinion, is the moral or valued way of thinking and acting, and hold on to your position."

Discussion Point: When a situation is dire, or lives are at stake, people might choose to give up their values. The problem is that borderline individuals often have black-and-white views on this issue: Either they are willing to sell out everything to get approval and liking (to give up their entire "self," it seems), or they interpret everything as an issue of values and view flexibility of any sort as giving up their integrity. Elicit examples.

4. **(be) T̲ruthful.** Explain: "Don't lie, act helpless when you are not, or exaggerate. A pattern of dishonesty over time erodes your self-respect. Even though one instance may not hurt, dishonesty as your usual mode of operating and getting what you want cannot fail to be harmful over the long run."

Acting helpless is the opposite of building mastery."

Discussion Point: At times, being honest may actually reduce relationship effectiveness. The "little white lie" was invented for just this reason. Any attempt to convince clients that honesty is *always* the best policy will probably fail. Discuss this point with participants. The crucial idea is that if one is going to lie, it should be done mindfully rather than habitually.

C. Self-respect effectiveness and objectives effectiveness.

Lecture Point: Explain: "It is important to remember that no one can take away your self-respect unless you give it up. Using **'DEAR MAN'** can improve self-respect by increasing a sense of mastery. So it is good to practice these skills. But you can also enhance self-respect by giving up things you want for the welfare of the other person. Using **'DEAR MAN'** effectively sometimes leads to a loss of self-respect for the other person. Balancing what you want and what the other person wants and needs might be the best path to self-respect."

D. Self-respect effectiveness and relationship effectiveness.

Lecture Point: Explain: "Most people's sense of self-respect is somewhat dependent on the quality of their relationships. Thus, using **'GIVE'** skills well will probably enhance your sense of self-respect. However, if you only use **'GIVE'** skills with a person who is abusive with you or doesn't care about you—always validating the other person, being interested, using an easy manner, and never threatening no matter what the other person does—your self-respect is likely to erode over time. Using **'GIVE'** skills when they are needed, and putting them away when harshness and boldness are necessary, might be the best path to self-respect."

XII. **Summarize** interpersonal goals; factors reducing effectiveness; cheerleading statements; and effectiveness skills for obtaining objectives, keeping relationships and keeping self-respect.

Notes

1. The importance of the wants-to-shoulds ratio was first discussed by Marlatt and Gordon (1985).

2. The wording here, while a bit awkward, is so that a "No" response to a question will mean "Say, no."

3. The idea for the four **DEAR** skills (describe, express, assert, reinforce) was taken from the "DESC scripts" (describe, express, specify, consequence) of Bower and Bower (1980). Their excellent self-help book is very compatible with DBT and can be used by both skills trainers and clients.

9

Emotion Regulation Skills

Borderline and suicidal individuals are emotionally intense and labile—frequently angry, intensely frustrated, depressed, and anxious. From a DBT perspective, difficulties in regulating painful emotions are central to the behavioral difficulties of the borderline individual. From the individual's perspective, painful feelings are most often the "problem to be solved." Suicidal behaviors and other dysfunctional behaviors, including substance abuse, are often behavioral solutions to intolerably painful emotions.

Their emotional intensity and lability suggest that borderline clients might benefit from help in learning to regulate their emotions. In my experience, most borderline individuals try to regulate emotions by instructing themselves not to feel whatever it is that they feel. This oversimplistic style is a direct result of the emotionally invalidating environment, which mandates that people should smile when they are unhappy, be nice and not rock the boat when they are angry, and confess and feel forgiven when they are feeling guilty.

Emotion regulation skills can be extremely difficult to teach, because a borderline individual has often been overdosed with remarks that if she would just "change her attitude" she could change her feelings. Many borderline individuals come from environments where everyone else exhibits almost perfect cognitive control of their emotions. Moreover, these very same others have exhibited both intolerance and strong disapproval of the individuals' inability to exhibit similar control. Often, borderline clients will resist any attempt to control their emotions, because such control would imply that other people are right and they are wrong for feeling the way they do. Thus, emotion regulation skills can be taught only in a context of emotional self-validation.

Like interpersonal effectiveness and distress tolerance, emotion regulation requires application of mindfulness skills—in this case, the nonjudgmental observation and description of one's current emotional responses. The theoretical idea is that much of the borderline individual's emotional distress is a result of secondary responses (e.g., intense shame, anxiety, or rage) to primary emotions. Often the primary emotions are adaptive and appropriate to the context. The reduction of this secondary distress requires exposure to the primary emotion in a nonjudgmental atmosphere. In this context, mindfulness to one's own emotional responses can be thought of as an exposure technique. (See Chapter 11 of the text for a fuller description of exposure-based procedures.) There are a number of specific DBT emotion regulation skills.

Specific Emotion Regulation Skills

Identifying and Labeling Emotions

The first step in regulating emotions is learning to identify and label current emotions. Emotions, however, are complex behavioral responses. Their identification often requires the ability not only to observe one's own responses but also to describe accurately the context in which the emotion occurs. Thus, learning to identify an emotional response is aided enormously if one can observe and describe (1) the event prompting the emotion; (2) the interpretations of the event that prompt the emotion; (3) the phenomenological experience, including the physical sensation, of the emotion; (4) the behaviors expressing the emotion; and (5) the aftereffects of the emotion on other types of functioning.

Identifying Obstacles to Changing Emotions

Emotional behavior is functional to the individual. Changing emotional behaviors can be extremely difficult when they are followed by reinforcing consequences; thus, identifying the functions and reinforcers for particular emotional behaviors can be useful. Generally, emotions function to communicate to others and to motivate one's own behavior. Emotional behaviors can also have two other important functions. The first, related to the communication function, is to influence and control other people's behaviors; the second is to validate one's own perceptions and interpretations of events. Although the latter function is not fully logical (e.g., if one person hates another, this does not necessarily mean that the other is worthy of being hated), it is nonetheless important for borderline individuals. Identifying these functions of emotions, especially negative emotions, is an important first step toward change.

Reducing Vulnerability to "Emotion Mind"

All people are more prone to emotional reactivity when they are under physical or environmental stress. Accordingly, the behaviors targeted here include balancing nutrition and eating, getting sufficient but not too much sleep (including treating insomnia if needed), getting adequate exercise, treating physical illness, staying off nonprescribed mood-altering drugs, and increasing mastery by engaging in activities that build a sense of self-efficacy and competence. The focus on mastery is very similar to activity scheduling in cognitive therapy for depression (Beck, Rush, Shaw, & Emery, 1979). Although these targets seem straightforward, making headway on them can be exhausting for both borderline clients and their therapists. With respect to insomnia, many of our borderline clients fight a never-ending battle in which pharmacotherapy often seems of little help. Poverty can interfere with both balanced nutrition and medical care. Work on any of these targets requires an active stance by the clients and persistence until positive effects begin to accumulate. The typical problem-solving passivity of many borderline individuals can create substantial interference here.

Increasing Positive Emotional Events

DBT assumes that most people, including borderline individuals, feel badly for good reasons. Although all people's perceptions tend to become distorted when they are highly emotional, that does not mean that the emotions themselves are the results of distorted perceptions. Thus, an important way to control emotions is to control the events that set off emotions. Increasing the number of pleasurable events in one's life is one approach to increasing positive emotions. In the short term, this involves increasing daily positive experiences. In the long term, it means making life changes so that pleasant events will occur more often. In addition to increasing positive events, it is also useful to work on being mindful of pleasurable experiences when they occur, as well as unmindful of worries that the positive experience will end.

Increasing Mindfulness to Current Emotions

Mindfulness to current emotions means experiencing emotions without judging them or trying to inhibit them, block them, or distract from them. The basic idea here is that exposure to painful or distressing emotions, without association to negative consequences, will extinguish their ability to stimulate secondary negative emotions. The natural consequences of a person's judging negative emotions as "bad" are feelings of guilt, anger, and/or anxiety whenever she feels distress. The addition of these secondary feelings to an already negative situation simply makes the distress more intense and tolerance more difficult. Frequently, the person could tolerate a distressing situation or painful affect if only she could refrain from feeling guilty or anxious about feeling painful emotions in the first place.

Taking Opposite Action

Behavioral-expressive responses are important parts of all emotions. Thus, one strategy to change or regulate an emotion is to change its behavioral-expressive component by acting in a way that opposes or is inconsistent with the emotion. This should include both overt actions (e.g., doing something nice for a person one is angry at, approaching what one is afraid of) and postural and facial expressiveness. With respect to the latter, however, clients must learn that the idea is not to block expression of an emotion; rather, it is to express a different emotion. There is a very big difference between a constricted facial expression that blocks the expression of anger and a relaxed facial expression that expresses liking.

Applying Distress Tolerance Techniques

Tolerating negative emotions without impulsive actions that make matters worse is, of course, one way to modulate the intensity and duration of negative emotions. Any or all of the distress tolerance techniques covered in the next chapter may be helpful; therefore, I do not discuss them here.

The instructional content of this module is divided into the following segments. The first segment deals with understanding the nature of emotions; a model of emotions provided and discussed. The second segment has to do with learning how to identify and label emotions in everyday life. The third segment focuses on identifying the functions of emotions and their relationship to difficulties in changing emotions. The fourth segment has to do with reducing vulnerability to negative emotions (emotion mind). The fifth segment deals with how to increase positive emotional events, and the sixth and final segment has to do with how to decrease emotional suffering through mindfulness to the current emotion and taking opposite action.

Content Outline

I. **Orient** clients to the skills to be learned in this module and the rationale for their importance.

> **Review Emotion Regulation Handout 1: Goals of Emotion Regulation Training.**

  A. **Understanding one's own emotions.**

   1. Learning to **identify emotions** as they are experienced: applying the mindfulness skills of observing and describing to emotions.

   2. Learning to identify what gets in the way of reducing intense negative emotions by analyzing the **functions of emotions**—the purposes they serve or needs they fulfill.

  B. **Reducing emotional vulnerability.**

   1. Learning to **decrease negative vulnerability**—to prevent negative emotional states by reducing the of likelihood of being overly emotionally sensitive (emotion mind) and increasing emotional hardiness.

   2. Learning to **increase positive emotions** and thus to reduce negative emotional sensitivity.

  C. **Decreasing emotional suffering.**

   1. Letting go of painful emotions by **being mindful to them,** instead of fighting them or walling them off.

   2. At times, modulating or changing a negative or painful emotion by acting **in a manner opposite to it.**

II. **Describe two kinds of emotional experiences.**

  A. Some emotional experiences are primarily reactions to events in one's environment (being angry at someone for criticizing, feeling happy that a loved one is coming to visit, being surprised that it is a nice day when rain was predicted, etc.).

  B. Other emotional experiences are primarily reactions to one's own thoughts, actions, and feelings (guilt about feeling angry, anger at being unable to remember something, shame at not doing well on a task, pride at winning a race, etc.).

  C. This module will focus on both kinds of emotions.

III. Describe the **role of emotions in people's lives.**

  A. Emotions can be useful or destructive, or (more rarely) neutral.

  Discussion Point: Elicit from participants when emotions have been useful and when they have been destructive. Have participants discuss the emotions that give them the most trouble. Which ones would they most like to work on?

  Note to Leaders: It is very important to get across the idea that the goal of emotion regulation is not to get rid of emotions or make people into zombies. Borderline individuals will always be emotional. The idea is to reduce their suffering. Determine which clients are afraid of losing all their emotions and which are trying to get rid of all their emotions.

  B. Appraisals of emotions—that is, what people say to themselves about emotions—can influence our ease and comfort with them.

  Lecture Point: A central problem for borderline individuals is that they react to most negative emotions with secondary emotions of guilt, shame, or anger. These secondary emotions cause all sorts of problems. In particular, they confuse the picture and make identification and description of the primary emotions very difficult. The primary emotions, are overshadowed by the secondary emotions; thus, problem solving in regard to the primary emotions is difficult. This topic will come up again and again in this module.

  Discussion Point: Elicit examples from participants of occasions when they have a secondary emotional reaction to a primary emotion (e.g., getting depressed about being depressed, getting angry or feeling ashamed for getting angry). Ask which usually causes them more trouble and pain—the primary or the secondary emotion?

> IV. **Review Emotion Regulation Handout 2: Myths about Emotions.**

  Discussion Point: Use the devil's advocate technique to discuss myths about emotions. The task of participants is to develop challenges or counterarguments to the myths. These challenges can be used as cheerleading statements later to help the clients feel better. Have everyone write challenges down as participants think them up.

Note to Leaders: See the discussion of Interpersonal Effectiveness Handout 4 in Chapter 8 of this manual (point VI in the content outline) for suggestions on using the devil's advocate strategy to discuss myths.

V. Present a **theory of emotions.**

A. There are probably about eight or so primary or basic emotions (e.g., anger, sorrow, joy, surprise, fear, disgust, guilt/shame, interest). People are born with the potential, or biological readiness, for these. All others are learned, and are usually some combination of the basic emotions.

B. Emotions are particular types of patterned reactions to events. They are complex and involve lots of components.

C. Emotions come and go. They are like waves in the sea. Most emotions only last from seconds to minutes.

D. Emotions are also self-perpetuating. Once an emotion starts, it keeps restarting itself. When an emotion seems to stay around, it is called a "mood."

E. Review Emotion Regulation Handout 3: Model for Describing Emotions.

Note to Leaders: Homework practice sheet for these skills is Emotion Regulation Homework Sheet 1: Observing and Describing Emotions. (The section on function is described later in the module, but is included in this homework sheet to cut down on the number of sheets.)

1. **Prompting event (inside or outside).** The events that prompt emotions can be outside in the environment, or they can be inside. A person's own thoughts, behaviors, and physical reactions can prompt emotions. One emotion can prompt another emotion. Some events can prompt emotions automatically; that is, a person can have an automatic reaction without any thoughts about the event. Fear when looking down from a high place is an example. Joy when looking at a beautiful sunset may be another example.

Discussion Point: Elicit other examples.

2. **Interpretation of event.** Most events do not automatically prompt emotions. Instead, the emotion is prompted by a person's interpretation of the event, or how the person appraises or thinks about the event.
   a. Example: Many fears are learned. People would not be afraid of guns if they did not believe that guns can kill.
   b. Example: Mary doesn't like Susan or Jenny. Susan gets very angry at Mary for not liking her; Jenny gets very afraid. Why? Susan is thinking how much she has done for Mary; Mary should appreciate it and like her. Jenny thinks that if Mary doesn't like her after all she has done for Mary, then maybe no one will like her.

Practice Exercise: Have participants think up events and interpretations that set off different emotions. One way to do this is to get one person to give a situation or event, have another give an interpretation, and have a third give the emotion. Then, for the same event, have a fourth person give another interpretation and a fifth figure out the emotion that would go with that interpretation. This can be repeated many times with the same event. Go through a number of events. The important point to make is that often people are responding to their own interpretations of an event, not to the event itself.

3. **Emotion:** Emotions are very complex, but generally consist of several parts or different reactions happening at the same time.
   a. Emotions involve **body changes,** such as tensing or relaxing of muscles, changes in blood vessels, fluctuations in heart rate, skin temperature, etc.
      i. The most important changes are in facial muscles. Researchers now think that changes in the facial muscles play a very important role in actually *causing* emotions.
      ii. Most people learn to inhibit or hide their body changes, at least some of the time. But even though the changes are not be obvious, very sensitive instruments could probably pick them up.

Discussion Point: Borderline individuals have learned better than most to hide their emotions by controlling the facial muscles that express emotions. This is a natural result of social learning in an emotionally invalidating environment. The hiding is usually automatic; that is, the individuals do not intend it or are not aware of it. This is a major reason why others often do not know that these persons are as upset as they are—they don't look it! Discuss how participants have learned to conceal their emotions in this way.

Discussion Point: It is also possible that a borderline individual is born with an emotional system that is less obviously expressive than the systems of others. It may be that this initial tendency to underexpress emotions (e.g., through facial expressions) sets up a situation where others in the environment do not get the feedback they need to monitor their interactions with the borderline individual appropriately. Thus, the environment becomes less responsive to emotional responses of the individual, setting up an invalidating pattern. Offer this hypothesis very tentatively and see how participants react to it.

    b. Emotions involve **brain changes.** Neurochemical changes in the brain are important parts of emotions. Some parts of the brain (e.g., the limbic system) appear to be very important in regulating emotions. The brain changes can then have effects on the rest of the body.

      i. Some researchers believe that one reason borderline individuals have trouble regulating emotions is that they have a problem in their brain chemistry.

      ii. Psychoactive drugs work to control emotions by changing brain chemistry. The problem is, however, that once the brain knows the drugs are there, it often changes the chemistry again to compensate for this.

    c. Emotions involve **sensing.** When people have emotional feelings, they are actually sensing their body and brain changes. This is usually what is meant by an "emotional experience."

Discussion Point: Explain: "Thus, when people tell you to quit feeling something, this is kind of silly. It would be like telling you to quit feeling the rain come down on your head. The only way to 'quit feeling' it is to divert your attention. Although that is sometimes easy to do, it is sometimes next to impossible. Telling a person with her foot in a burning fire to divert her attention would be kind of silly." Discuss this idea.

Practice Exercise: Lead participants in a series of exercises where they try to quit feeling/sensing something (e.g., their arms on their chair arms), and then try diverting their attention. Explain: "Sometimes the problem in emotions is that you cannot sense your body and body changes. To regulate emotions, you have to be pretty good at sensing your body. If you have been

practicing shutting off all sensations for years, this can be difficult."

Discussion Point: Get feedback on which clients have difficulty sensing their bodies and which have difficulty pin-pointing exactly what part of their bodies they are sensing. Discuss the notion that for some people, emotions are like a fog; they can't see (sense) what exactly an emotion is.

    d. Emotions involve **action urges.** An important function of emotions is to prompt behavior (e.g., fight in anger, flight in fear). Although the action itself is usually not considered part of the emotion, the urge to act is.

Discussion Point: Discuss action urges of several emotions. Elicit feedback from participants.

    e. In the case of very complex emotions, **interpretations, beliefs, and assumptions** may be part of the emotions. For example, despair is sadness combined with a belief that things are terrible and will not get better.

4. **Expression.** One of the most important functions of emotions is to communicate. If it is to do that, an emotion has to be expressed.

    a. The expression of primary or basic emotions is "hard-wired" into human beings. Research shows that in all cultures, the same facial expressions are linked to the same basic emotions. Many actions that express emotions are also hard-wired.

    b. People can learn to inhibit emotional expressions or to express them differently. For complex emotions that are learned, the expressions are learned.

    c. Different facial expressions and behaviors may express different emotions, depending on one's overall culture, regional culture (e.g., the South vs. the Northwest in the United States), our family culture, school culture, and individual differences.

Discussion Point: Discuss the fact that each family, town, state, etc., is a miniculture. Expressiveness that is OK in one miniculture, may not be OK in another. Get examples from participants' own experience.

Discussion Point: Discuss the point that what an expression means can vary from time to time and person to person. Thus, reading emotions is easy in some senses but very difficult. People often misread one another's emotions. The same behavior can express many different emotions. The same emotion can be expressed by many different behaviors. Discuss when participants have been misread and have misread others.

    5. **Types of expression.**
        a. Body language (e.g., postural and facial changes).
        b. Words (e.g., "I love you," "I hate you," "I am sad," "I'm sorry").
        c. Actions (kissing, hitting, running toward someone, withdrawing passively, avoiding, doing cartwheels).
    6. **Emotion name.** Every culture gives names to emotions. There is some evidence that people who can give an emotion a name are better able to control the emotion. How to name emotions is learned. Obviously, it is easier to name simple emotions than complex ones.

VI. Present the concept of **recognizing, describing, and naming emotions.**
    A. Describing an emotion involves describing:
        1. **Prompting events** and situation.
        2. **Interpretation** of the event or situation (i.e., thoughts, assumptions, beliefs).
        3. **Body responses** that are sensed (or can be sensed if one pays attention).
        4. **Body language,** (i.e., face and posture).
        5. **Verbal communication** of the emotion.
        6. **Action urges** and actions taken.

Lecture Point: By learning to observe your emotions, you learn to be separate from (not identified as) your emotions and also at one with your emotions. In order to control, you must be separate from your emotions so that you can think and use coping strategies. But you also need to be one with your emotions, in the sense that you identify them as part of yourself and not something outside you. Give the example of a horse and rider: To the extent that the rider is "one" with her horse she can control the horse. If she is separate, fighting the horse, the horse will fight back and she cannot control it smoothly. On the other hand, if the rider is mindless, so to speak, and has no identity separate from the horse, she will just cling to the horse for dear life and the horse will assume all direction.

    B. Emotions also have **aftereffects.**

Lecture Point: Intense emotions have powerful aftereffects on memory, thoughts, and even the ability to think, physical function and behavior. In a sense, we can say **"emotions love themselves."** They organize the person in such a way as to continue (or keep refiring) the very same emotion.

Lecture Point: Explain: "These are typical emotion words and typical features or characteristics of emotions. Much of the handout was made up by ordinary people in response to questions about their emotional experiences."

Note to Leaders: The primary intent of this handout is to give clients ideas when they have trouble describing characteristics of their own emotions. It does not have to be gone over in detail. You might just flip through it, explaining what it is, and have clients read it between sessions. Some will find this very helpful, others not so helpful. It is essential not to convey that the features listed on the handout are necessary to each emotion. These are typical features, but because of culture and individual learning, features may differ from person to person.

Discussion Point: Have participants give their own ideas about characteristics of emotions.

Practice Exercise: Have clients engage in role-play practice.
    1. Have each person think of an emotional situation to role-play.
    2. Give instructions in how to do role-play. Have two clients role-play the situation, or you can role-play it with one client. Have everyone observe the situation, and describe nonverbal expressive behavior of the role-play participants. Guide clients to pay special attention to faces.
    3. Have the role players describe how they felt and what they were expressing.

Note to Leaders: See Chapter 8 of this manual (point X in the content outline) for further suggestions regarding the conduct of role-playing practice.

VII. Describe **factors that interfere with observing and describing emotions.**
    A. **Secondary emotions** (emotional reactions to emotions). As noted earlier, when a secondary emotion comes on the scene, it can cover up or confuse the primary emotional reaction.
    B. **Ambivalence** (more than one emotional reaction to the same event).

Note to Leaders: These points are usually best made during homework sharing. Participants should fill out as many homework sheets (Emotion Regulation Homework Sheet 1) as there are prompting events. Thus, if a person has a secondary emotional reaction prompted by the original emotion or set of emotions, she should fill out a second homework sheet. You need to be particularly vigilant about this during homework sharing; it can be very difficult to sort out.

VIII. Review Emotion Regulation Handout 5: What Good Are Emotions?

Note to Leaders: Homework practice sheet for these skills is Emotion Regulation Homework Sheet 2: Emotion Diary.

A. Why do people have emotions? Many animals have emotional behaviors. Emotional behavior is very immediate and efficient. In fact, it is probably necessary for survival.

B. If there were no function or need for emotions, they would be easy to change. But because they have a purpose (serve a need, etc.), they can be very hard to change.

C. **Emotions communicate to (and influence) others.**

   1. Facial expressions are a hard-wired part of emotions. In primitive societies and among animals, facial expressions communicate like words. Even in modern societies, facial expressions communicate faster than words.

      a. Having both verbal and nonverbal forms of emotional expression means having two ways of communication for important situations.

      b. Some emotional expressions have an automatic effect on others. That is, the effect is not learned.

         i. For example, an infant reacts spontaneously to an adult's smile or look of fright. This automatic reaction serves infants well until they learn to use words. Even after they can use words, facial expressions are still very helpful.

         ii. When body expressions of emotion (facial, posture, voice tone) and what a person says don't go together, other people almost always will trust the nonverbal expressions over the verbal ones.

Discussion Point: This is a very important point. A major premise of DBT is that one of the problems of borderline individuals is that their nonverbal emotional

expressions are often not accurate indicators of what the individual is experiencing, and thus they are often misread. Get examples from participants of being misread or of misreading others because of mismatched nonverbal communication.

   2. When it is important to communicate to others, or send them a message, it can be very hard to change emotions.

      a. Example: If Jane wants Kathy to know that Kathy is in the wrong, then Jane may want to remain angry until Kathy gets the message. If Jane stops being angry, Kathy may not take her seriously or may not realize that she is indeed in the wrong.

      b. Example: If Julie wants Emily to realize how dangerous the situation they are in is, Julie may not want to stop being afraid. Otherwise, Emily may think the situation is safe.

      c. If Maria wants Terry to know what she likes, she may want to stay joyful.

   3. The communication of emotions influences others, whether a person intends it or not.

      a. Examples: Warmth and friendliness of an acquaintance may result in a later favor; disappointment expressed by a supervisor may result in improved work by an employee; anger may result in one person's giving another her rightful due instead of withholding it.

      b. Example: Feeling worthless, hopeless, and agonizingly sad may influence a therapist or another person to take away the pain. (So the hope goes.)

      c. Example: Expressed anger may stop others' behavior.

Discussion Point: Get participants to give examples of their emotions' influencing others and of their being influenced by others' emotions, and discuss. Also, elicit examples of times when this strategy boomeranged—that is, when participants' expression of emotion got them something they didn't want.

Discussion Point: Elicit communication value of guilt/shame, surprise, love, and sadness, as well as of the emotions mentioned in examples above.

D. **Emotions organize and prepare for action.**

   1. Emotions prepare for and motivate behavior. The action urge connected to specific emotions is hard-wired.

   2. This saves time in getting people to act in

important situations. They don't have to think everything through.

    a. Example: In communities where there is no sadness at losing people, why would anyone ever go out and look for lost people or try to save people who are dying? Communities would die off if there were no sadness.

    b. Example: Students often do not want to reduce test anxiety because they are afraid that if they do, so they will quit working so hard and then fail their tests.

    c. Example: People are afraid to reduce guilt because they are afraid that without guilt they will start doing harmful things.

Discussion Point: Elicit and discuss other examples, especially examples having to do with anger.

E. For humans, emotions also function to **communicate to ourselves.** Emotions can be **"self-validating."**

1. People often use their emotional reactions to other people and to events as information about the situation. Emotions can be signals or alarms that something is going on.

    a. This is what is meant by the saying "Pay attention to (or listen to) your gut."

    b. Likewise, when we say a person has a "good feel for a situation," we are referring to emotions as signals.

    c. Sometimes signals picked up from the situation at a nonconscious (or automatic) level are processed. This processing sets off an emotional reaction, but the person cannot identify what about the situation set off the emotion. Through trial and error—that is, experience—people learn when to trust these emotional responses as information about the situation, and when to believe that they are providing information about the persons responding rather than about the situation.

Discussion Point: Get examples from participants of when their "feel" for a situation proved to be correct. Discuss how people often ignore their own "sense" or "feel" for a situation simply because they can't put into words good reasons for that "sense," or because other people disagree.

Note to Leaders: Note that using one's emotions this way is the same as using the countertransference to give you a clue about your clients. That is, therapists are often trained to use emotions in this way.

2. When this use of emotions is carried to an extreme, emotions are treated as facts: "If I feel incompetent, I am." "If I get depressed when left alone, I shouldn't be left alone." "If I feel right about something, it is right." People use their emotions to tell themselves that what they believe is correct.

Note to Leaders: This issue is both crucial and very sensitive for borderline individuals. A primary function of negative emotions for them is self-validation. This is understandable once you remember the invalidating environments most have experienced. The way it works is as follows: When a person's feelings are minimized or invalidated, then it is difficult for her to get her concerns and needs taken seriously. Also, too much may be asked or expected of her. One way to counteract this is for her to increase the intensity of her emotions. Sooner or later, she will probably be attended to. If then at a later point the person does not get very emotional under the same circumstances, then it proves other people right: Her emotions weren't valid in the first place. After enough of these instances, the person's integrity is on the line with her emotions. If the situation is not as bad as she says it is, then she is shameful for having caused so much trouble to others. *Ergo,* the function of negative emotions gradually evolves to that of self-validation. Getting these points across to borderline individuals is fraught with difficulty because the very idea is invalidating. Care, patience, and skill are needed here.

Discussion Point: Get participants to give examples and discuss. Draw from them instances where emotions are self-validating and where changing negative emotions is invalidating. Give personal examples if you can think of any.

  IX. **Prepare to present methods** for reducing emotional vulnerability

A useful way to remember these skills is the phrase **"PLEASE MASTER."**

Treat **P**hysica**l** illness
Balance **E**ating
Avoid Mood-**A**ltering drugs
Balance **S**leep
Get **E**xercise

Build **MASTER**y

> X. **Review Emotion Regulation Handout 6: Reducing Vulnerability to Negative Emotions: How to Stay out of Emotion Mind.**

> **Note to Leaders:** Homework practice sheet for these skills is Emotion Regulation Homework Sheet 3: Steps for Reducing Painful Emotions. Some skills are also included on the back of the DBT diary card.

A. **Treat Physical illness.** Explain: "Being sick lowers your resistance to negative emotions."

Discussion Point: Discuss any illnesses participants have had. What interferes with treating illness? Embarrassment about the problem (as in the case of sexually transmitted diseases), lack of assertion skills, and lack of money are common obstacles.

B. **Balance Eating.** Explain: "Try to eat the amounts and kinds of foods that help you feel good—not too much or too little."

Discussion Point: Discuss the research on restrained eaters that shows the negative effects of eating too little. The idea is also for people to stay away from foods that make them feel bad. Stress avoiding these. Ask participants for foods that make them feel good (e.g., chocolate), calm (e.g., milk), or energized (e.g., sugar, meat); stress the role of such foods, in moderation.

C. **Avoid mood-Altering drugs.** Explain: "Alcohol and drugs, like certain foods, can lower resistance to negative emotions."

Discussion Point: Use this as an opportunity to discuss alcohol and drug problems participants may be having. Discuss effects of drugs on emotions, as well as difficulties in staying off mood-altering drugs.

D. **Balance Sleep:** Explain: "Try to get the amount of sleep that helps you feel good—not too much or too little."

Discussion Point: Elicit participants' troubles with sleep. This is usually an important problem for borderline individuals. Too little sleep, especially, can make them particularly vulnerable to negative emotions; it may be part of a depression syndrome. What has helped? What has made things worse?

E. **Get Exercise.** Explain: "Aerobic exercise, done consistently, is an antidepressant. In addition, a regular exercise schedule can build mastery."

Discussion Point: Ask what forms of exercise participants are engaging in. An important problem here is that consistent exercise requires self-management skills, and most borderline individuals have few such skills. This discussion is an opportunity to discuss principles of self-management, especially reinforcement principles.

F. **Build MASTERy.** Explain: "Do things that make you feel competent, self-confident, in control, and capable of mastering things."

Lecture Point: Doing things to build mastery is an important component of cognitive therapy for depression, which is a very effective therapy. The idea is to build a sense of confidence and competence. Doing so makes a person more resistant to depression and other negative emotions. Building mastery usually requires doing something that is at least a little bit hard or challenging.

Discussion Point: Elicit activities that give participants a sense of mastery. These will probably differ for each person.

> **XI. Review Emotion Regulation Handout 7: Steps for Increasing Positive Emotions.**

A. **Building positive experiences.** Explain: "Increase the number of events that prompt positive emotions, such as love, joy, pride, self-confidence, and calm."

Note to Leaders: As noted earlier, a basic point in DBT is that most people, including borderline individuals, who feel painful emotions do so for good reasons. The assumption here is that it is usually (but not always) the events in life that cause unhappiness, not faulty appraisals of events. This is pretty much the opposite of what is assumed by many therapists. A reconciliation between the two points of view is possible, however. Once a person gets emotional, she distorts; thus, vigilance for distorting is useful, and reappraisal can be helpful. However, focusing on cognitive distortions as the source of difficulty simply further invalidates the behavior, emotions, and thinking processes of the borderline individual. Instead, the goal is to *validate* the individual's responses.

1. **Short term.** Explain: "Do pleasant things that are possible now. Increase daily positive experiences."

> **Note to Leaders:** Give out Emotion Regulation Handout 8: Adult Pleasant Events Schedule. Encourage clients to do as many as possible of those things on the schedule that make them feel happy or joyful.

Discussion Point: Elicit little things that participants find pleasant. Be creative. Get some ideas from the "Crisis Survival Strategies" handout (Distress Tolerance Handout 1; see Chapter 10 of this manual).

2. **Long term.** Explain: "Make changes in your life so that positive events will occur more often."

   a. Explain: "Make a list of positive events you want in your life. These are your goals. **Work toward these goals.**"

Lecture Point: No one is very happy if she doesn't have many positive events in her lives. This is a basic point of DBT. It is hard to be happy without a life worth living. Building a life worth living—one that is satisfying and one that brings happiness—is like saving pennies in a piggy bank. A person has to accumulate positives.

   b. Explain: **"Attend to relationships.** Repair old relationships. Make new relationships."

Lecture Point: Most people need good relationships to be happy. Many people are not very happy unless they are in one or more close relationships. Explain: "The secret here is not to put all your eggs in one basket. Don't let your entire happiness depend on one person or one group (for example, a romantic relationship, your family)."

   c. Explain: **"Avoid avoiding.** Avoid giving up."

Lecture Point: No one can build up a positive life if she avoids problem solving or doing things that are necessary.

B. **Mindfulness of positive experience.** Explain: "Be mindful of positive events that occur. Do the following:

   1. Focus your attention on positive events that happen.
   2. Refocus on positive parts of events when your mind wanders to the negative."

C. **Unmindfulness of worries.** Explain: "Do not destroy positive experiences. Be unmindful of the following:

   1. Thinking about when it will end.
   2. Thinking about whether you deserve it.
   3. Thinking about how much is expected of you now."

Lecture Point: These are extremely important skills. Many borderline individuals can experience positive emotions, but these evaporate in a second; they do not last. Thus, clients have to work really hard at learning how to get positive emotions to linger. Often they are afraid that if they feel good, bad things will happen—that is, they have a phobia of positive emotions. Or a negative thought intrudes quickly. These points should be stressed.

XII. Review Emotion Regulation Handout 9: Letting Go of Emotional Suffering: Mindfulness of Your Current Emotion.

A. **Mindfulness of emotions** means observing and describing them just as they are.

   1. Explain: "This strategy is useful because it allows you to get distance from your emotions. Distance is crucial for figuring things out and for problem solving in regard to emotions."
   2. Observing emotions is a form of **exposure.** It works on the same principle that exposure does in treating fear and panic. Explain: "By exposing yourself to emotions, but not necessarily acting on them, you will find that they are not so catastrophic. You will stop being so afraid of them. Once you are less afraid, all the fear, panic, anger, and so forth that result from your emotions' being as they are will dissipate."

B. The best way to get rid of negative and painful emotions is to **let them go.** But learning to let go is extremely difficult.

C. Letting go of emotions is not the same as pushing them away. Fighting pain usually makes it worse.

Lecture Point: Painful emotions are part of the human condition. Once again, DBT assumes that there are valid reasons for negative emotions. Short of making tremendous life changes, people probably cannot get rid of a lot of them; even then, negative emotions will always be a part of life. *Ergo,* the trick is to find a new way of relating to negative emotions so that they do not induce so much suffering. The way is through acceptance. Accepting painful emotions eliminates the suffering, leaving only the pain. At times, acceptance even reduces the pain. Fighting emotions insures that they stay. This is simply a restatement of the principles of mindfulness (see Chapter 7 of this manual) and of distress tolerance (see Chapter 10), but these points are extremely important to get across.

Discussion Point: Discuss the role of acceptance and emotional suffering. Usually, you can expect borderline individuals to get this point. Get feedback.

D. Explain: "The basic steps in letting go are as follows:

   1. Observe your emotion. Acknowledge its presence. Step back. Get unstuck from the emotion.
   2. Try to experience your emotion as a wave,

coming and going. (It can be very useful here to concentrate on *just* physical parts of the emotion, or *just* quality of experience, or the like.)

Try not to block or suppress the emotion. Open yourself to the flow of the emotion.

Do not try to get rid of the emotion. Don't push it away. Don't judge or reject it.

Do not try to keep the emotion around. Don't cling to it. Don't rehearse it. Don't hold on to it. Don't amplify it.

3. Note that you are *not* your emotion.

Do not necessarily act on the emotion.

4. Trying to build a wall to keep emotions out always has the effect of keeping emotions in. Instead, practice loving your your emotions. Be willing to have them."

Lecture Point: This last point is of course a difficult one. "Loving" in this context means "acceptance." Fighting emotions does not make them go away. Accepting emotions allows a person to do something about them. Refer to the example of the horse and rider (see item VI, above). The idea of loving and accepting emotions also does not mean increasing or augmenting them.

Story Point: The following story is adapted from one I was told by a Zen teacher, who read it in a book by another spiritual teacher, Anthony de Mello, S.J., (1983). The story is a very helpful one in teaching the concept of loving one's emotions.

A man bought a new house and decided that he was going to have a very beautiful lawn. He worked on it every week, doing everything the gardening books told him to do. His biggest problem was that the lawn always seemed to have dandelions growing where he didn't want them. The first time he found dandelions, he pulled them out. But, alas, they grew back. He went to his local gardening store and bought weed killer. This worked for some time, but after summer rains, alas, he found dandelions again. He worked and pulled and killed dandelions all summer. The next summer he thought he would have no dandelions at all, since none grew over the winter. But, then, all of a sudden, he had dandelions all over again. This time he decided the problem was with the type of grass. So he spent a fortune and had all new sod put down. This worked for some time and he was very happy. Just as he started to relax, a dandelion came up. A friend told him it was due to the dandelions in the lawns of his neighbors. So he went on a campaign to get all his neighbors to kill all their dandelions. By the third year, he was exasperated. He still had dandelions. So, after consulting every local expert

and garden book, he decided to write the U.S. Department of Agriculture for advice. Surely the government could help. After waiting several months, he finally got a letter back. He was so excited. Help at last! He tore open the letter and read the following: "Dear Sir: We have considered your problem and have consulted all of our experts. After careful consideration, we think we can give you very good advice. Sir, our advice is that you learn to love those dandelions."

This story can be told as often as necessary. The idea is to get to the point where clients say to you, "I know, this is a dandelion."

Discussion Point: Have participants share times when radical acceptance of emotions has reduced suffering. Share your own experiences. Discuss the idea of "loving" one's emotions.

Practice Exercise: Have participants fill out Homework Sheet 1 or 2 ("Observing and Describing Emotions" or "Emotion Diary"). Discuss the emotion they have selected and what events set it off.

E. Explain: "**Respect your emotion.** Don't assume that it is irrational or based on faulty perceptions or distortions."

XIII. Review Emotion Regulation Handout 9: Changing Emotions by Acting Opposite to the Current Emotion.

Lecture Point: Some psychotherapy researchers believe that when treatments for emotional disorders work, they do so because they reverse the expressive and action components of emotional responses. For example, a number of researchers have observed that effective therapies for depression all share a common thread: They activate behavior. Similarly, effective therapies for anxiety disorders all share a common thread of nonreinforced exposure to feared situations. Effective treatments for anger tend to stress learning to identify the cues to frustration and/or anger and leaving the situation. It is essential to get across to clients the rationale for this technique and to elicit their cooperation. See the section on exposure-based procedures in Chapter 11 of the text for a more extensive discussion.

A. **Fear.** Explain: "When you are afraid, approach what you are afraid of rather than avoid it. Do what you are afraid to do rather than avoid it."

B. **Guilt or shame.** Explain: "When you are guilty or ashamed, keep doing what you feel guilty or ashamed of (assuming that the guilt is unjustified). Again, approach, don't avoid. When you are guilty or ashamed and the emotion is justified by your behavior, repair the situation, apologize, and then go on."

C. **Sadness or depression.** Explain: "When you are depressed, get active. Do things that make you feel competent and self-confident rather than acting passive. Again, approach, don't avoid."

D. **Anger.** Explain: "When you are angry, gently avoid the person you are angry with rather than attacking. (This means also avoiding thinking about him or her rather than ruminating.) Distract yourself: Do something nice rather than mean. Try to be sympathetic rather than blaming."

Lecture Point: It is very important to note that the idea here is to act contrary to an emotion, not to mask or hide emotions. Explain: "You have to throw your entire self into acting opposite to the emotion. But you do not have to suppress your feelings. Your behavior or actions communicate to your brain, and the effect is a slow but steady change in your emotions. This procedure works when your emotions are not realistic for the situation. Thus, if the problem is fear, you should only enter fearful situations if there is no serious danger. If the problem is guilt or shame, don't repeat actions that in your wise mind you believe are immoral."

Practice Exercise: Have participants pay attention to sensations in their faces. Guide them in noting any areas of tension. Now instruct each person to imagine a situation during the past week when she felt angry or sad or worried. While she is thinking about it, she should again notice sensations in the face. Instruct participants to raise a hand slightly to signal to you when they have the situation in mind. Now, as they continue to imagine, instruct them to try to mask the feelings so that no one else in the room (if anyone was looking) would know the feeling or even realize that feelings exist. Have them notice the sensations in the face; have them notice what happens to the emotions. Next, instruct each person to relax her facial muscles, smoothing them out as much as she can. Have participants notice how emotions change (or don't change); have them notice how different the face feels. It is common for clients to report that when they relax their faces, they feel much more vulnerable. Explain: "This means you are allowing feelings to come and go. You are not holding them in or pushing them out."

Practice Exercise: The very best practice exercises are those in which you can get participants to act differently from how they feel right in the group. Over and over during modules, look for opportunities to instruct members to do their best to not act in accord with their emotions of the moment. For example, when clients want to leave out of anger, anxiety, hurt feelings, or panic, instruct them to stay, orienting them to how staying is practicing acting opposite to their emotions. Periodically, as, "What do you do when you are afraid?" Coach them until they can always chime out, "Do what you are afraid of!" "What do you do when you're depressed?" "Get active!" "What do you do when you feel guilty?" "Figure out if it is justified and either repair it or do it over and over and over (if not)!" And so on. Drill members until they have this cold.

XIV. **Summarize** emotion regulation goals, emotion myths, observing and describing emotions, function or purpose of emotions, reducing vulnerability to negative emotions, increasing vulnerability to positive emotions, mindfulness to the current emotion, and acting opposite to the current emotion.

10

Distress Tolerance Skills

Goals of the Module

Most approaches to mental health treatment focus on changing distressing events and circumstances. They have paid little attention to accepting, finding meaning for, and tolerating distress. Although the distinction is not as clear-cut as I am making it seem, this task has generally been tackled by religious and spiritual communities and leaders. DBT emphasizes learning to bear pain skillfully. The ability to tolerate and accept distress is an essential mental health goal for at least two reasons. First, pain and distress are part of life; they cannot be entirely avoided or removed. The inability to accept this immutable fact itself leads to increased pain and suffering. Second, distress tolerance, at least over the short run, is part and parcel of any attempt to change oneself; otherwise, impulsive actions will interfere with efforts to establish desired changes.

Distress tolerance skills constitute a natural progression from mindfulness skills. They have to do with the ability to accept, in a nonevaluative and nonjudgmental fashion, both oneself and the current situation. Essentially, distress tolerance is the ability to perceive one's environment without putting demands on it to be different, to experience your current emotional state without attempting to change it, and to observe your own thoughts and action patterns without attempting to stop or control them. Although the stance advocated here is a nonjudgmental one, this should not be understood to mean that it is one of approval. It is especially important that this distinction be made clear to clients: Acceptance of reality is not equivalent to approval of reality.

The distress tolerance behaviors targeted in DBT skills training are concerned with tolerating and surviving crises and with accepting life as it is in the moment. Four sets of crisis survival strategies are taught: distract-ing, self-soothing, improving the moment, and thinking of pros and cons. Acceptance skills include radical acceptance (i.e., *complete* acceptance from deep within), turning the mind toward acceptance (i.e., *choosing* to accept reality as it is), and willingness versus willfulness. Gerald May (1982) describes willingness as follows:

> Willingness implies a surrendering of one's self-separateness, an entering into, an immersion in the deepest processes of life itself. It is a realization that one already is a part of some ultimate cosmic process and it is a commitment to participation in that process. In contrast, willfulness is the setting of oneself apart from the fundamental essence of life in an attempt to master, direct, control, or otherwise manipulate existence. More simply, willingness is saying yes to the mystery of being alive in each moment. Willfulness is saying no, or perhaps more commonly, "yes, but . . . " (p. 6)

Although borderline clients and their therapists alike readily accept crisis survival skills as important, the DBT focus on acceptance and willingness is often viewed as inherently flawed. This viewpoint is based on the notion that acceptance and willingness imply approval. This is not what May means; indeed, he points out that willingness demands opposition to destructive forces, but goes on to note that it seems almost inevitable that this opposition often turns into willfulness:

> But willingness and willfulness do not apply to specific things or situations. They reflect instead the underlying attitude one has toward the wonder of life itself. Willingness notices this wonder and bows in some kind of reverence to it. Willfulness forgets it, ignores it, or at its worst, actively tries to destroy it. Thus willingness can sometimes seem very active and assertive, even aggressive. And willfulness can appear in the guise of passivity. Political revolution is a good example. (p. 6)

Content Outline

I. **Orient** clients to skills to be learned in this module and the rationale for their importance.

   A. **Skills for tolerating and surviving crises.**

   B. **Skills for accepting life as it is in the moment.**

Lecture Point: The skills in the module are ones that help people get through life when they can't make changes for the better in their situation and when, for any number of reasons, they can't sort out their feelings well enough to make changes in how they feel. Basically, the skills are ways of surviving and doing well in terrible situations without resorting to behaviors that will make the situations worse.

Discussion Point: Everyone has to tolerate some amount of pain and distress in life. Life simply is not pain-free. Always trying to avoid pain leads to more problems than it solves. Get examples from participants of this point.

Lecture Point: Present the research literature on avoidance. Posttraumatic stress disorder is primarily a result of trying to avoid all contact with cues that cause discomfort. Pathological grieving—that is, grieving that never ends—is a result of the same avoidance. Avoiding all cues that are associated with pain insures that the pain will continue. The more people attempt to avoid and shut emotional (as well as physical) pain off, the more it comes back to haunt them. Trying to suppress emotional pain or avoid contact with pain-related cues leads to ruminating about the painful events; paradoxically, trying to get rid of painful thoughts creates painful thoughts. For example, one of the most successful and effective programs for helping people with chronic physical pain is based almost entirely on the practice of mindfulness and is described in the book *Full Catastrophe Living* by Jon Kabat-Zinn (1990). (See also the section on exposure-based treatments in Chapter 11 of the text.) Experiencing, tolerating, and accepting emotional pain are the ways to reducing pain.

Lecture Point: But there are times for people to distract themselves from pain also. Painful situations cannot always be immediately processed. It is often not an appropriate time for working on painful emotions or situations. At work, at school, or at meetings, people may feel emotional pain, be upset, or feel alienated. However, they may simply have to tolerate the feelings. This module is not about working things out or changing things; it is about accepting and tolerating things.

Discussion Point: Elicit examples of times when pain is intense but it is not an appropriate time to work on changing the source of the pain or figuring out and changing the painful emotions. Discuss the relationship of this module to the fact that not much time in skills training is spent processing feelings.

> II. **Review Distress Tolerance Handout 1: Crisis Survival Strategies.**

> **Note to Leaders:** Homework practice sheet for these skills is Distress Tolerance Homework Sheet 1: Crisis Survival Strategies.

   A. Give **overview** of skills.

   1. The skills to be learned here are concrete skills in how to tolerate and survive a crisis situation when the crisis cannot be changed right away.

   2. The basic idea is to learn how to get through bad situations without making them worse.

Discussion Point: Elicit from participants crisis situations they need to tolerate.

Discussion Point: Surviving crisis situations is part and parcel of being effective, "doing what works" (a core mindfulness skill). However, at times people are more interested in proving to others how bad a situation is than in surviving the situation. The problem with proving how bad things are is that it hardly ever works. That is, although it may result in short-term gains (e.g., being put in the hospital or getting a lover to return), it usually fails in the long run. Elicit situations where this has been the case with clients. Leaders: If you can give personal examples here, so much the better.

   3. There are four categories of crisis survival strategies: distracting, self-soothing, improving the moment, and focusing on pros and cons. Each is a series of methods for short-circuiting or coping with overwhelming negative emotions and intolerable situations.

   4. These strategies are intended for getting through crisis situations and overwhelming emotions. They are not presented as a cure all for one's problems or life. Beneficial effects may only be temporary (but achieving them is not a small feat, nonetheless). Remind participants that these are not presented as emotion regulation strategies (i.e., ways to reduce or end painful emotions), although they may help to regulate emotions. They are, instead, ways to survive painful emotions.

Discussion Point: Get participants to discuss where and why such strategies might be a good idea. That is, why is surviving a crisis a good idea? Pull for insight that temporary solutions are at times OK.

B. Review **specific skills.**

1. **Distracting** methods have to do with reducing contact with emotional stimuli (events that set off emotions). Or, in some cases, they work to change parts of an emotional response. There are seven distracting skills. A useful way to remember these skills is the phrase **"Wise Mind ACCEPTS":**

> <u>A</u>ctivities
> <u>C</u>ontributing
> <u>C</u>omparisons
> <u>E</u>motions
> <u>P</u>ushing away
> <u>T</u>houghts
> <u>S</u>ensations

a. <u>**Activities**</u> can work to modulate negative emotions in a number of ways. They distract attention and fill short-term memory with thoughts, images, and sensations counteractive to the thoughts, images, and sensations that activate and reactivate the negative emotion. They affect physiological responses and emotional expressive behavior directly.

b. <u>**Contributing**</u> refocuses attention from oneself to what one can do for others. For some, contributing also increases a sense of meaning in life, thereby improving the moment (see below). For others, it also enhances self-respect.

c. Making <u>**Comparisons**</u> also refocuses attention from oneself to others, but in a different way. In this case, the situations of others—those coping in the same way or less well, or the less fortunate in general—are used to recast one's own situation in a more positive light.

d. Generating opposite <u>**Emotions**</u> replaces the current negative emotion with other, less negative emotions. This strategy interferes with the current mood state. This technique requires the person to first figure out the current emotion so that activities to generate an opposite one can be sought.

e. <u>**Pushing away**</u> from a situation can be done by leaving it physically or by blocking it in one's mind. Leaving the situation decreases contact with the emotion-

al cues associated with the situation. Blocking is a somewhat conscious effort to inhibit internal stimuli associated with negative emotions. Blocking is a bit like riding a bicycle; one only understands it when one does it. (Most borderline clients seem able to do this and will usually know what you mean as soon as you mention the technique.) It is perhaps related to the ability to dissociate or depersonalize. It should not be the first technique tried, but can be useful in an emergency. The secret is not to overuse it.

f. Distracting with other <u>**Thoughts**</u> fills short-term memory with other thoughts so that thoughts activated by the negative emotion do not continue to reactivate the emotion.

g. Intense other <u>**Sensations**</u> can interfere with the physiological component of the current negative emotion. Also, the sensations may work to focus attention on something other than the stimuli arousing the emotion. Holding ice cubes,[2] in particular, can be very helpful. In a skills group of a colleague of mine, a client brought everyone small refreezable ice packs. Several clients would then take them (frozen) to therapy sessions to hold onto when discussing very painful topics (e.g., sexual abuse that one client had not previously been able to discuss at all). This latter technique, while at times useful, would also need to be closely monitored so that it does not interfere with exposure to important and relevant cues.

Discussion Point: Elicit any objections participants have to using distraction, and discuss. Cheerleading may be needed.

2. **Self-soothing** has to do with comforting, nurturing, and being gentle and kind to oneself. A way to remember these skills is to think of soothing each of the **Five senses:**

> <u>**Vision**</u>
> <u>**Hearing**</u>
> <u>**Smell**</u>
> <u>**Taste**</u>
> <u>**Touch**</u>

Note to Leaders: The meaning and intent of these

are reasonably self-evident, so you need to review only a few in session. You should devote more time to the following discussion point.

Discussion Point: Borderline individuals often have difficulties with self-soothing. Some believe that they do not deserve soothing, kindness, and gentleness; they may feel guilty or ashamed when they self-soothe. Others believe that they should get soothing from others; they don't self-soothe as a matter of principle, or feel angry at others when they attempt to self-soothe. Elicit examples from each participant.

Note to Leaders: It is important that each participant learn to self-soothe. Even if at first it elicits anger or guilt, self-soothing should be repeatedly attempted. In time, it will become easier. Some clients may be quite resistant to practicing self-soothing. Keep a watchful eye on homework practice to be sure that each participant is at least trying these skills. Assess and problem-solve difficulties.

3. **Improving the moment** is replacing immediate negative events with more positive ones. Some strategies for improving the moment are cognitive techniques having to do with changing appraisals of oneself (encouragement) or the situation (positive thinking, meaning, imagining). Some involve changing body responses to events (relaxing). Prayer and focusing on one thing in the moment have to do with acceptance and letting go. A way to remember these skills is the word **"IMPROVE:"**

> I̱magery
> M̱eaning
> P̱rayer
> Ṟelaxation
> O̱ne thing in the moment
> V̱acation
> E̱ncouragement

a. **I̱magery** can be used to distract, soothe, bolster courage and confidence, and make future rewards more salient. Explain: "Using imagery, you can create a situation different from the actual one; in this sense, it is like leaving the situation. With imagery, however, you can be sure that the place you go to is a safe and secure one. Going to an imaginary safe place or room within can be very helpful during flashbacks. For it to be useful, however, you have to practice it when you are not in a crisis enough times to get it firmly down as a skill."

Imagery can also be used to cope more effectively with crises. Practicing effective coping in imagination can actually increase one's chances of coping with it effectively in real life.

b. Finding or creating **M̱eaning** helps many people in crises. Victor Frankl (1984) wrote an important book about surviving Nazi concentration camps, *Man's Search for Meaning,* based on the premise that people need to find or create meaning in their lives to survive terrible suffering. Finding or creating meaning is similar to the dialectical strategy of making lemonade out of lemons. (See Chapter 7 of the text.)

Discussion Point: It is important to note that life is at times unfair for reasons that no one can understand. People do not have to assume that there is a purpose to their suffering, although those who are religious or spiritual may see it this way. Those who do not believe in a higher purpose can still create meaning or purpose, however. Get feedback about participants' views on the meaning or purpose of suffering.

c. The essence of **P̱rayer** is the complete opening of oneself to the moment. This practice is very similar to the notion of radical acceptance, discussed later in this module. Note that the suggested prayer is not one of begging to have the suffering or crisis taken away. Nor is it a "Why me?" prayer.

Practice Exercise: During the skills training session, have all participants close their eyes, imagine or "get in touch with" a current pain or suffering, and then silently try each type of prayer (an acceptance prayer, a "Deliver me" prayer, a "Why me?" prayer). Have participants refocus on current suffering (for only a moment) before each attempt at prayer. Discuss afterwards. Or suggest that people who are comfortable with praying try each type of prayer during the next crisis and keep track of which type actually helps.

d. **Ṟelaxing** is changing how the body responds to stress and crises. Often people tense their bodies as if by keeping them tense, they can actually make the situation change. They try to control the situation by controlling their bodies. The goal here is to accept reality with the body. The idea is that the body communicates with the mind, accepting with the body can help in accepting with the mind.

Note to Leaders: Most clients who have been on an inpatient psychiatric unit will have gotten muscle relaxation training. Check on how they liked it and whether it was useful. You may also want to do some structured relaxation training here; any of the numerous audio-tapes available for this can be used. It is important to point out that relaxing is a skill that takes lots of practice. The breath and half-smiling exercises described below are relaxation exercises that promote acceptance and tolerance. They are specific and concrete, and both can be done in crisis situations. Practiced on a daily basis, they can prepare clients for crises.

e. **One thing in the moment** is the second mindfulness "how" skill discussed in Chapter 7 of this manual. Although it can be very difficult to do, focusing on one thing in the moment can be very helpful in the middle of a crisis; it can provide time to settle down. The secret of this skill is to remember that the only pain one has to survive is "just this moment." We all often suffer much more than is required by calling to mind past suffering and ruminating about future suffering we may have to endure. But, in reality, there is only "just this moment." Because of the importance of this skill in reality acceptance, a number of specific exercises for improving focus and increasing awareness are taught in the next section of this module.

Practice Exercise: During the session, have all participants close their eyes and imagine or "get in touch with" some current discomfort, irritation, or anxiety right now, this moment in the session. Instruct participants to raise a hand slightly when they have the focus. Instruct them to notice their level of current discomfort. Now instruct them to start ruminating about all the past times they have had to endure such feelings in sessions. Have them also bring to mind and ruminate about how much more of these feelings have to be endured in this skills training session and all future sessions. Instruct them to notice now their level of discomfort. Then have them refocus the mind on "just this moment." Explain: "Say in your mind 'just this moment.' Let go of thoughts of the future and the past." Have them notice now their level of discomfort. Discuss the exercise.

f. Taking a "**Vacation** from adulthood" is ceasing to cope actively and either retreating into oneself or allowing oneself to be taken care of for the moment. Explain: "Everyone needs a vacation from adulthood once in a while. The trick is to take it in a way that does not harm you, and also to make sure the vacation is brief. It should only last from a few moments to no longer than a day. When you have responsibilities, taking a vacation depends on getting someone else to take over your duties for a while." The idea here is similar to Alan Marlatt's (Marlatt & Gordon, 1985) use of planned relapses in the treatment of addictions. The focus is on the *planned* nature of the relapse (or, here, the *planned* vacation). It is similar to the notion of taking a timeout to regroup.

Discussion Point: Borderline individuals are usually experts at taking vacations. The problem is that they are not in control of their vacations; that is, they take them at inappropriate times and stay on them too long. Making vacation taking a skill to be practiced, gives them the potential for getting in control. Elicit from participants times they have taken vacations in an out-of-control fashion. Discuss ways to get in control of vacations and use them effectively.

g. **Encouragement** is cheerleading oneself. Explain: "The idea is to talk to yourself as you would talk to someone you care about who is in a crisis. Or talk to yourself as you would like someone else to talk to you." Leaders: You may at first need to do quite a bit of modeling here, as well as cheerleading.

4. **Thinking of pros and cons** consists of thinking about the positive and negative aspects of tolerating distress and the positive and negative aspects of not tolerating it. The eventual goal here is for the person to face the fact that accepting reality and tolerating distress lead to better outcomes than do rejecting reality and refusing to tolerate distress.

Practice Exercise: Many borderline individuals react to crises and stress by harming themselves (parasuicidal behavior, substance abuse, "throwing tantrums," etc.). Make a "pros" column and a "cons" column on the blackboard. Get participants to generate pros and cons of tolerating a crisis without doing something harmful and/or impulsive. Then generate a list of pros and cons for not tolerating the crisis (for self-harm, substance abuse, or one or more other nontolerating responses the participants want to analyze). Be sure to focus on both short-term and long-term pros and cons. Compare the two sets of lists.

5. **Notes/Other Ideas** is a space at the end of Handout 1 to write down ideas that participants generate for tolerating distress. Almost always, clients will have a number of creative strategies not on the list. Write these ideas down and ask other participants to do so.

Discussion Point: Discuss with participants how these strategies can be overused in invalidating environments. Point out that the fact that they can be overused does not mean they have no value at all. Elicit and problem-solve "resistance" to using these skills.

III. Go over **breath, half-smiling, and awareness exercises.**

Note to Leaders: If you are running short of time, give the general idea of each of these exercises, but let participants read and practice each specific one on their own. For those who find these exercises helpful, suggest that they read the book *The Miracle of Mindfulness* by Thich Nhat Hanh (1976). These exercises are drawn from that book.[3] It is very important that leaders also practice these skills.

> **A. Review Distress Tolerance Handout 2: Guidelines for Accepting Reality: Observing-Your-Breath Exercises.**

Lecture Point: All major religions and spiritual disciplines have as an important part of their contemplative and/or meditative practice a focus on breathing. The focus is intended to help the individuals accept and tolerate themselves, the world, and reality as it is. A focus on breathing is also an important part of relaxation training and the treatment of panic attacks.

1. Go over one or several breath exercises (using guidelines):
   a. Deep breathing.
   b. Measuring your breath by your footsteps.
   c. Counting your breath.
   d. Following your breath while listening to music.
   e. Following your breath while carrying on a conversation.
   f. Following the breath.
   g. Breathing to quiet the mind and body.
2. Have each participant select one breath exercise she would like to try during the coming week.

> **B. Review Distress Tolerance Handout 3: Guidelines for Accepting Reality: Half-Smiling Exercises.**

1. Explain: "Half smiling is accepting and tolerating with your body. To do it, you relax your face, neck, and shoulder muscles, and then half-smile with your lips. Try to adopt a serene facial expression. Remember to *relax* the facial muscles." (See Chapter 11 of text and Chapter 9, this manual, for further discussion.)

Lecture Point: Emotions are partially controlled by facial expressions. By adopting a half-smile—a serene, accepting face—people can control their emotions somewhat. They can feel more accepting if their faces express acceptance.

2. Go over one or more half-smiling exercises (using guidelines):
   a. Half-smile when you first awake in the morning.
   b. Half-smile during your free moments.
   c. Half-smile while listening to music.
   d. Half-smile when irritated.
   e. Half-smile in a lying down position.
   f. Half-smile in a sitting position.
   g. Half-smile while contemplating the person you hate or despise the most.

Practice Exercise: Have participants sit very still. First, have them try to make a very impassive face—one with no expression—and experience how that feels. Then have them try actually relaxing the muscles of the face—from the forehead, to the eyes, to the cheeks, and to the mouth and jaw—and experience how that feels. Finally, have them half-smile and experience how that feels. Discuss the differences.

3. Have each participant select one half-smiling exercise she would like to try during the coming week.

> **C. Review Distress Tolerance Handout 4: Guidelines for Accepting Reality: Awareness Exercises.**

Lecture Point: These exercises can be very helpful in the middle of a crisis. When practiced every day, they can help develop a more accepting state of mind.

1. Go over one of several awareness exercises (using guidelines):
   a. Awareness of the positions of the body.
   b. Awareness of connection to the universe.
   c. Awareness while making tea or coffee.
   d. Awareness while washing the dishes.
   e. Awareness while hand-washing clothes.
   f. Awareness while cleaning house.

g. Awareness while taking a slow-motion bath.

h. Practicing awareness with meditation.

2. Have each participant select an awareness exercise she would like to try during the coming week.

Note to Leaders: Do not underestimate the value of these awareness exercises for getting through very difficult times. In truly desperate times, these can be exceptionally valuable. In my experience, almost all borderline individuals like and use these—at least if you first push them to give them a try. Notice that one could make up any number of variations.

> **IV. Review Distress Tolerance Handout 5: Basic Principles of Accepting Reality.**

> **Note to Leaders:** Homework practice sheet for these skills and the remaining skills in this module is Distress Tolerance Homework Sheet 2: Acceptance and Willingness.

A. **Radical acceptance** is letting go of fighting reality. The term "radical" means to imply that the acceptance has to come from deep within and has to be complete. Acceptance is the only way out of hell. It is the way to turn suffering that cannot be tolerated into pain that can be tolerated. Pain is part of living; it can be emotional and it can be physical. Pain is nature's way of signaling that something is wrong, or that something needs to be done.

1. The pain of a hand on a hot stove causes a person to move her hand quickly. People without the sensation of pain are in deep trouble.

2. The pain of grief causes people to reach out for others who are lost. Without it there would probably be no societies or cultures. No one would look after those who are sick, would search for loved ones who are lost, or would stay with people who are difficult at times.

3. Pain of fear makes people avoid what is dangerous.

4. Pain of anger makes people overcome obstacles.

Discussion Point: What are the pros and cons of never having painful emotions? Would participants like people who never have painful emotions?

Lecture Point: Suffering is pain plus nonacceptance of the pain. Suffering comes when people are unable or refuse to accept pain. Suffering comes when people cling to getting what they want, refusing to accept what they have. Suffering comes when people resist reality as it is at the moment. Pain can be difficult or almost impossible to bear, but suffering is even more difficult. Refusal to accept reality and the suffering that goes along with it can interfere with reducing pain. It is like a cloud that surrounds pain, interfering with the ability to see it clearly. Radical acceptance transforms suffering to pain.

Discussion Point: When acceptance is used as a technique to create change—as a sort of "bargain with God" ("I'll accept it, and in return you promise to make it better")—is not really acceptance. Elicit examples of bargaining from participants.

Note to Leaders: The point of radical acceptance is extremely difficult for borderline individuals (and some leaders) to see. They have great difficulty seeing that they can accept something without approving of it. They believe that if they accept what is, they cannot change it. Trying to get them to accept the notion of acceptance, can become a power struggle. As a shaping strategy, you might suggest the terms "acknowledge," "recognize," or "endure." Discuss these points. You will probably have to discuss them over and over again. Great patience is needed, but don't give up on radical acceptance.

Discussion Point: A great myth is that if people don't accept something, if they simply refuse to put up with it, it will magically change. It is as if resistance and/or willpower alone, will change it. Get examples of this. Discuss why participants might believe this. Elicit examples of when tantrums and verbal refusals to accept things have been reinforced.

Discussion Point: Some people are afraid that if they ever actually accept their painful situation or emotions, they will become passive and just give up (or give in). Elicit and discuss fears of participants. Explain: "Imagine that you hate the color purple. Then imagine that your room is painted purple. If you refuse to accept that the room is purple, you will never paint it a color you want." Elicit examples of when accepting things as they are has helped to reduce suffering and resulted in a greater ability to reduce the source of pain. (This point is taken up again below under willingness versus willfulness.)

Discussion Point: The notion of acceptance is central to every major religion, East and West. Elicit participants' reactions to this and any experiences they have. The idea is also similar to the Alcoholics Anonymous notion of surrendering to a higher power and accepting things one cannot change.

B. **Turning the mind** is choosing to accept. Acceptance seems to require some sort of choice. People have to turn their minds in that direction, so to speak. Acceptance sometimes only lasts a moment or two, so people have to keep turning the mind over and over and over. The choice has to be made every day—sometimes many, many times a day, or even an hour or a minute.

Discussion Point: Discuss all the reasons why *not* to accept, to turn the mind. Elicit reasons from participants. What makes it so difficult to take that first step?

C. The notion of **willingness versus willfulness** is taken from Gerald May's (1982) book on the topic.

1. **Willingness** is accepting what is, together with responding to what is, in an effective or appropriate way. It is doing what works. It is doing just what is needed in the current situation or moment.

2. **Willfulness** is imposing one's will on reality—trying to fix everything, or refusing to do what is needed. It is the opposite of doing what works.

Lecture Point: Use metaphors to explain willingness versus willfulness. One is that life is like hitting baseballs from a pitching machine. A person's job is just to do her best to hit each ball as it comes. Refusing to accept that a ball is coming does not make it stop coming. Willpower, defiance, crying, or whimpering does not make the machine stop pitching the balls; they keep coming over and over and over. A person can stand in the way of a ball and get hit, stand there doing nothing and let the ball go by as a strike, or swing at the ball. Another metaphor is that life is like a game of cards. It makes no difference to a good card player what cards she gets. The object is to play whatever hand she gets as well as possible. As soon as one hand is played, another hand is dealt. The last game is over and the cur-

rent game is on. The idea is to be mindful of the current hand, play it as skillfully as possible, and then let go and focus on the next hand of cards. Many other metaphors (e.g., life as a computer game) can be used also.

Discussion Point: Elicit examples of willingness and willfulness. Leaders: If you can point to recent examples of yourselves' and/or participants' being willful or willing, so much the better. A light touch is needed. Discuss May's definitions. Elicit agreements and disagreements.

Practice Exercise: The best way to get the ideas of willingness and willfulness off the written page and into active use is to start highlighting during skills training sessions when you (the leaders) and/or the clients are behaving willfully and when willingly. Phrase it as a question: "Do you all think I am being willful here? Hmmm, let's examine this," or "You're not by chance being willful about this, are you?" (Clients will usually rather enjoy catching the leaders in willfulness.) Or when a difficult situation or conflict emerges in a session, you can say, "OK. Let's all try to be completely willing for the next 5 minutes."

V. **Summarize** rationale for distress tolerance, crisis survival strategies, radical acceptance, willingness and willfulness.

Notes

1. R. Matthew Kamins, Cornell Medical Center/New York Hospital at White Plains, made very helpful comments about how to reorganize these skills.

2. Steve Hollon of Vanderbilt University gave me this idea.

3. Distress Tolerance Handouts 2, 3, and 4 are adapted from *The Miracle of Mindfulness: A Manual on Meditation* (pp. 79–87, 93) by Thich Nhat Hanh, 1976, Boston: Beacon Press. Copyright 1976 by Thich Nhat Hanh. Adapted by permission.

References

Barley, W. D., Buie, S. E., Peterson, E. W., Hollingsworth, A. S., Griva, M., Hickerson, S. C., Lawson, J. E., & Bailey, B. J. (in press). The development of an inpatient cognitive-behavioral treatment program for borderline personality disorder. *Journal of Personality Disorders.*

Beck, A. T., Rush, A. J., Shaw, B. F., & Emery, G. (1979). *Cognitive therapy of depression.* New York: Guilford Press.

Borkovec, T. D., & Inz, J. (1990). The nature of worry in generalized anxiety disorder: A predominance of thought activity. *Behaviour Research and Therapy, 28,* 153–158.

Bower, G., & Bower, S. (1980). *Asserting yourself: A practical guide for positive change.* Reading, MA: Addison-Wesley.

Chamberlain, P. Patterson, G., Reid, J., Kavanagh, K., & Forgatch, M. (1984). Observation of client resistance. *Behavior Therapy, 15,* 144–155.

de Mello, A., S. J., (1993). *The song of the bird.* Anand, India: Gujarat Sahitya Prakash.

Deikman, A. J. (1982). *The observing self: Mysticism and psychotherapy.* Boston: Beacon Press.

Frankl, V. E. (1984). *Man's search for meaning: An introduction to logotherapy* (3rd ed.). New York: Simon & Schuster.

Goldberg, C. (1980). The utilization and limitations of paradoxical intervention in group psychotherapy. *International Journal of Group Psychotherapy, 30,* 287–297.

Hanh, T. N. (1976). *The miracle of mindfulness: A manual on meditation.* Boston: Beacon Press.

Kabat-Zinn, J. (1990). *Full catastrophe living: Using the wisdom of your body and mind to face stress, pain, and illness.* New York: Dell.

Linehan, M. M. (1993). *Cognitive behavioral treatment for borderline personality disorder.* New York: Guilford Press.

Linehan, M. M., Armstrong, H. E., Suarez, A., Allmon, D., & Heard, H. L. (1991). Cognitive–behavioral treatment of chronically parasuicidal borderline patients. *Archives of General Psychiatry, 48,* 1060–1064.

Linehan, M. M., Goldfried, M. R., & Goldfried, A. P. (1979). Assertion therapy: Skill training or cognitive restructuring. *Behavior Therapy, 10,* 372–388.

Linehan, M. M., & Heard, H. L. (1993). Impact of treatment accessibility on clinical course of parasuicidal patients. In reply to R. E., Hoffman [Letter to the editor]. *Archives of General Psychiatry, 50,* 157–158.

Linehan, M. M., Heard, H. L., & Armstrong, H. E. (in press). Naturalistic follow-up of a behavioral treatment for chronically suicidal borderline patients. *Archives of General Psychiatry.*

Linehan, M. M., & Koerner, K. (1992). Behavioral theory of borderline personality disorder. In J. Paris (Ed.), *Handbook of borderline personality disorder.* Washington, DC: American Psychiatric Press.

Linehan, M. M., Sharp, E., & Ivanoff, A. M. (1980). *The Adult Pleasant Events Schedule.* Paper presented at the meeting of the Association for Advancement of Behavior Therapy, New York.

Maccoby, E. E. (1980). *Social development.* New York: Harcourt Brace & Jovanovich.

Marlatt, G. A., & Gordon, J. R. (Eds.). (1985). *Relapse prevention: Maintenance strategies in the treatment of addictive behaviors.* New York: Guilford Press.

May, G. (1982). *Will and spirit.* San Francisco: Harper & Row.

The original Oxford English dictionary on computer disc (Version 4.10) [Computer file]. (1987). Fort Washington, PA: Tri Star.

Patterson, G. R., & Forgatch, M. S. (1985). Therapist behavior as a determinant for client noncompliance: A paradox for the behavior modifier. *Journal of Consulting and Clinical Psychology, 53,* 846–851.

Polanyi, M. (1958). *Personal knowledge.* Chicago: University of Chicago Press.

Shaver, P., Schwartz, J., Kirson, D., & O'Connor, C. (1987). Emotion knowledge: Further exploration of a prototype approach. *Journal of Personality and Social Psychology, 52,* 1061–1086.

Handouts and Homework Sheets

EMOTION REGULATION HANDOUTS

EMOTION REGULATION HOMEWORK SHEETS

DISTRESS TOLERANCE HANDOUTS

DISTRESS TOLERANCE HOMEWORK SHEETS

Note to Leaders: Two-page Handouts and Homework Sheets will be much easier to use if copied back-to-back. Clients should be given several copies of each Homework Sheet. Handouts can be copied on 3-hole-punch paper and given to clients in a 3-ring binder.

GENERAL HANDOUT I

Goals of Skills Training

GENERAL GOAL

To learn and refine skills in changing behavioral, emotional, and thinking patterns associated with problems in living, that is, those causing misery and distress.

SPECIFIC GOALS

Behaviors to Decrease

1. Interpersonal chaos

2. Labile emotions, moods

3. Impulsiveness

4. Confusion about self, cognitive dysregulation

Behaviors to Increase

1. Interpersonal effectiveness skills

2. Emotion regulation skills

3. Distress tolerance skills

4. Core mindfulness skills

From *Skills Training Manual for Treating Borderline Disorder Personality* by Marsha Linehan. ©1993 The Guilford Press.

GENERAL HANDOUT 2

Guidelines for Skills Training

1. Clients who drop out of therapy are out of therapy.

2. Each client has to be in ongoing individual therapy.

3. Clients are not to come to sessions under the influence of drugs or alcohol.

4. Clients are not to discuss past (even if immediate) parasuicidal behaviors with other clients outside of sessions.

5. Clients who call one another for help when feeling suicidal must be willing to accept help from the persons called.

6. Information obtained during sessions, as well as the names of clients, must remain confidential.

7. Clients who are going to be late or miss a session should call ahead of time.

8. Clients may not form private relationships outside of skills training sessions.

9. Sexual partners may not be in skills training together.

Other Rules for this Group/Notes:

_____

_____

_____

_____

_____

_____

_____

_____

From *Skills Training Manual for Treating Borderline Disorder Personality* by Marsha Linehan. ©1993 The Guilford Press.

MINDFULNESS HANDOUT 1

Taking Hold of Your Mind:

States of Mind

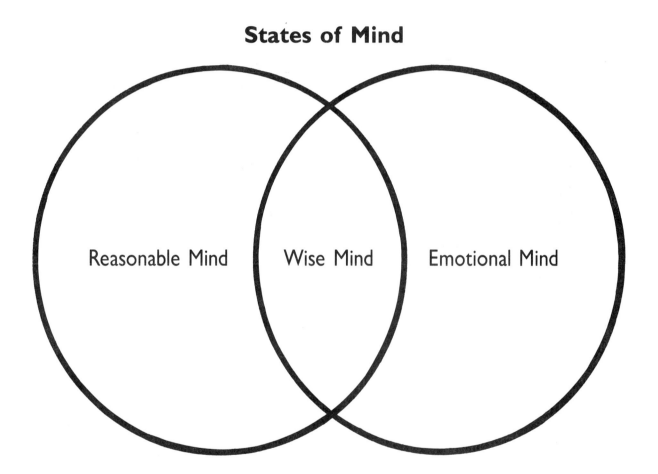

Reasonable Mind   Wise Mind   Emotional Mind

MINDFULNESS HANDOUT 2

Taking Hold of Your Mind: "What" Skills

OBSERVE

- JUST NOTICE THE EXPERIENCE. Notice without getting caught in the experience. Experience without reacting to your experience.

- Have a "TEFLON MIND," letting experiences, feelings, and thoughts come into your mind and slip right out.

- CONTROL your attention, but not what you see. Push away nothing. Cling to nothing.

- Be like a guard at the palace gate, ALERT to every thought, feeling, and action that comes through the gate of your mind.

- Step inside yourself and observe. WATCH your thoughts coming and going, like clouds in the sky. Notice each feeling, rising and falling, like waves in the ocean. Notice exactly what you are doing.

- Notice what comes through your SENSES—your eyes, ears, nose, skin, tongue. See others' actions and expressions. "Smell the roses."

DESCRIBE

- PUT WORDS ON THE EXPERIENCE. When a feeling or thought arises, or you do something, acknowledge it. For example, say in your mind, "Sadness has just enveloped me." . . . or . . . "Stomach muscles tightnening" . . . or . . . "A thought 'I can't do this' has come into my mind." . . . or . . . "walking, step, step, step. . . . "

- PUT EXPERIENCES INTO WORDS. Describe to yourself what is happening. Put a name on your feelings. Call a thought just a thought, a feeling just a feeling. Don't get caught in content.

PARTICIPATE

- Enter into your experiences. Let yourself get involved in the moment, letting go of ruminating. BECOME ONE WITH YOUR EXPERIENCE, COMPLETELY FORGETTING YOURSELF.

- ACT INTUITIVELY from wise mind. Do just what is needed in each situation—a skillful dancer on the dance floor, one with the music and your partner, neither willful nor sitting on your hands.

- Actively PRACTICE your skills as you learn them until they become part of you, where you use them without self-consciousness. PRACTICE:

    1. Changing harmful situations.
    2. Changing your harmful reactions to situations.
    3. Accepting yourself and the situation as they are.

From *Skills Training Manual for Treating Borderline Personality Disorder* by Marsha Linehan. ©1993 The Guilford Press.

MINDFULNESS HANDOUT 3

Taking Hold of Your Mind: "How" Skills

NON-JUDGMENTALLY

- See but DON'T EVALUATE. Take a nonjudgmental stance. Just the facts. Focus on the "what," not the "good" or "bad," the "terrible" or "wonderful," the "should" or "should not."

- UNGLUE YOUR OPINIONS from the facts, from the "who, what, when, and where."

- ACCEPT each moment, each event as a blanket spread out on the lawn accepts both the rain and the sun, each leaf that falls upon it.

- ACKNOWLEDGE the helpful, the wholesome, but don't judge it. Acknowledge the harmful, the unwholesome, but don't judge it.

- When you find yourself judging, DON'T JUDGE YOUR JUDGING.

ONE-MINDFULLY

- DO ONE THING AT A TIME. When you are eating, eat. When you are walking, walk. When you are bathing, bathe. When you are working, work. When you are in a group, or a conversation, focus your attention on the very moment you are in with the other person. When you are thinking, think. When you are worrying, worry. When you are planning, plan. When you are remembering, remember. Do each thing with all of your attention.

- If other actions, or other thoughts, or strong feelings distract you, LET GO OF DISTRACTIONS and go back to what you are doing—again, and again, and again.

- CONCENTRATE YOUR MIND. If you find you are doing two things at once, stop and go back to one thing at a time.

EFFECTIVELY

- FOCUS ON WHAT WORKS. Do what needs to be done in each situation. Stay away from "fair" and "unfair," "right" and "wrong," "should" and "should not."

- PLAY BY THE RULES. Don't "cut off your nose to spite your face."

- Act as SKILLFULLY as you can, meeting the needs of the situation you are in. Not the situation you wish you were in; not the one that is just; not the one that is more comfortable; not the one that. . . .

- Keep an eye on YOUR OBJECTIVES in the situation and do what is necessary to achieve them.

- LET GO of vengeance, useless anger, and righteousness that hurts you and doesn't work.

From *Skills Training Manual for Treating Borderline Disorder Personality* by Marsha Linehan. ©1993 The Guilford Press.

INTERPERSONAL EFFECTIVENESS HANDOUT 1

Situations for Interpersonal Effectiveness

ATTENDING TO RELATIONSHIPS

- Don't let hurts and problems build up.
- Use relationship skills to head off problems.
- End hopless relationships.
- Resolve conflicts before they get overwhelming.

BALANCING PRIORITIES vs. DEMANDS

- If overwhelmed, reduce or put off low-priority demands.
- Ask others for help; say no when necessary.
- If not enough to do, try to create some structure and responsibilities; offer to do things.

BALANCING THE WANTS-TO-SHOULDS

- Look at what you do beçause you enjoy doing it and "want" to do it; and how much you do because it has to be done and you "should" do it. Try to keep the number of each in balance, even if you have to:
  - Get your opinions taken seriously.
  - Get others to do things.
  - Say no to unwanted requests.

BUILDING MASTERY AND SELF-RESPECT

- Interact in a way that makes you feel competent and effective, not helpless and overly dependent.
- Stand up for yourself, your beliefs and opinions; follow you own wise mind.

From *Skills Training Manual for Treating Borderline Disorder Personality* by Marsha Linehan. ©1993 The Guilford Press.

INTERPERSONAL EFFECTIVENESS HANDOUT 2

Goals of Interpersonal Effectiveness

OBJECTIVES EFFECTIVENESS:
Getting Your Objectives or Goals in a Situation

- Obtaining your legitimate rights
- Getting another to do something
- Refusing an unwanted or unreasonable request
- Resolving an interpersonal conflict
- Getting your opinion or point of view taken seriously

QUESTIONS

1. *What specific results or changes do I want from this interaction?*
2. *What do I have to do to get the results? What will work?*

RELATIONSHIP EFFECTIVENESS:
Getting or Keeping a Good Relationship

- Acting in such a way that the other person keeps liking and respecting you
- Balancing immediate goals with the good of the long-term relationship

QUESTIONS

1. *How do I want the other person to feel about me after the interaction is over?*
2. *What do I have to do to get (or keep) this relationship?*

SELF-RESPECT EFFECTIVENESS:
Keeping or Improving Self-Respect and Liking for Yourself

- Respecting your own values and beliefs; acting in a way that makes you feel moral
- Acting in a way that makes you feel capable and effective

QUESTIONS

1. *How do I want to feel about myself after the interaction is over?*
2. *What do I have to do to feel that way about myself? What will work?*

From *Skills Training Manual for Treating Borderline Personality Disorder* by Marsha Linehan. ©1993 The Guilford Press.

INTERPERSONAL EFFECTIVENESS HANDOUT 3

Factors Reducing Interpersonal Effectiveness

LACK OF SKILL

You actually DON'T KNOW what to say or how to act. You don't know how you should behave to achieve your objectives. You don't know what will work.

WORRY THOUGHTS

Worry thoughts get in the way of your ability to act effectively. You have the ability, but your worry thoughts interfere with doing or saying what you want.

- WORRIES ABOUT BAD CONSEQUENCES.
  "They won't like me," "She will think I am stupid."
- WORRIES ABOUT WHETHER YOU DESERVE TO GET WHAT YOU WANT.
  "I am such a bad person I don't deserve this."
- WORRIES ABOUT NOT BEING EFFECTIVE AND CALLING YOURSELF NAMES.
  "I won't do it right," "I'll probably fall apart," "I'm so stupid."

EMOTIONS

Your emotions (ANGER, FRUSTRATION, FEAR, GUILT) get in the way of your ability to act effectively. You have the ability, but your emotions make you unable to do or say what you want. Emotions, instead of skill, control what you say and do.

INDECISION

You CAN'T DECIDE what to do or what you really want. You have the ability, but your indecision gets in the way of doing or saying what you want. You are ambivalent about your priorities. You can't figure out how to balance:

- Asking for too much versus not asking for anything.
- Saying no to everything versus giving in to everything.

ENVIRONMENT

Characteristics of the environment make it impossible for even a very skilled person to be effective. SKILLFUL BEHAVIOR DOESN'T WORK.

- Other people are too powerful.
- Other people will be threatened or have some other reason for not liking you if you get what you want.
- Other people won't give you what you need or let you say no without punishing you unless you sacrifice your self-respect, at least a little.

From *Skills Training Manual for Treating Borderline Disorder Personality* by Marsha Linehan. ©1993 The Guilford Press.

INTERPERSONAL EFFECTIVENESS HANDOUT 4

Myths about Interpersonal Effectiveness

1. I can't stand it if someone gets upset with me.

   CHALLENGE: _____

2. If they say no, it will kill me.

   CHALLENGE: _____

3. I don't deserve to get what I want or need.

   CHALLENGE: _____

4. If I make a request, this will show that I am a very weak person.

   CHALLENGE: _____

5. I must be really inadequate if I can't fix this myself.

   CHALLENGE: _____

6. I have to know whether a person is going to say yes before I make a request.

   CHALLENGE: _____

7. Making requests is a really pushy (bad, self-centered, selfish, un-christian) thing to do.

   CHALLENGE: _____

8. It doesn't make any difference; I don't care really.

   CHALLENGE: _____

9. Obviously, the problem is just in my head. If I would just think differently I wouldn't have to bother everybody else.

   CHALLENGE: _____

10. This is a catastrophe (is really bad, is terrible, is driving me crazy, will destroy me, is a disaster).

    CHALLENGE: _____

11. Saying no to a request is always a selfish thing to do.

    CHALLENGE: _____

12. I should be willing to sacrifice my own needs for others.

    CHALLENGE: _____

13. _____

    CHALLENGE: _____

14. _____

    CHALLENGE: _____

From *Skills Training Manual for Treating Borderline Personality Disorder* by Marsha Linehan. ©1993 The Guilford Press.

INTERPERSONAL EFFECTIVENESS HANDOUT 5

Cheerleading Statements
for Interpersonal Effectiveness

1. It is OK to want or need something from someone else.

2. I have a choice to ask someone for what I want or need.

3. I can stand it if I don't get what I want or need.

4. The fact that someone says no to my request doesn't mean I should not have asked in the first place.

5. If I didn't get my objectives, that doesn't mean I didn't go about it in a skillful way.

6. Standing up for myself over "small" things can be just as important as "big" things are to others.

7. I can insist on my rights and still be a good person.

8. I sometimes have a right to assert myself, even though I may inconvenience others.

9. The fact that other people might not be assertive doesn't mean that I shouldn't be.

10. I can understand and validate another person, and still ask for what I want.

11. There is no law that says other people's opinions are more valid than mine.

12. I may want to please people I care about, but I don't have to please them all the time.

13. Giving, giving, giving is not the be-all of life. I am an important person in this world, too.

14. If I refuse to do a favor for people, that doesn't mean I don't like them. They will probably understand that, too.

15. I am under no obligation to say yes to people simply because they ask a favor of me.

16. The fact that I say no to someone does not make me a selfish person.

17. If I say no to people and they get angry, that does not mean that I should have said yes.

18. I can still feel good about myself, even though someone else is annoyed with me.

OTHERS: _____

_____

_____

_____

From *Skills Training Manual for Treating Borderline Personality Disorder* by Marsha Linehan. ©1993 The Guilford Press.

INTERPERSONAL EFFECTIVENESS HANDOUT 6

Options for Intensity of Asking or Saying No, and Factors to Consider in Deciding

OPTIONS

HIGH INTENSITY: TRY AND CHANGE THE SITUATION

Ask firmly, insist... **6** ...Refuse firmly, don't give in.

Ask firmly, resist no... **5** ...Refuse firmly, resist giving in.

Ask firmly, take no... **4** ...Refuse firmly, but reconsider.

Ask tentatively, take no... **3** ...Express unwillingness.

Hint openly, take no... **2** ...Express unwillingness, but say yes.

Hint indirectly, take no... **1** ...Express hesitancy, say yes.

Don't ask, don't hint... **0** ...Do what other wants without being asked.

LOW INTENSITY: ACCEPT THE SITUATION AS IT IS

FACTORS TO CONSIDER

1. PRIORITIES: OBJECTIVES very important? Increase intensity.
RELATIONSHIP very tenuous? Consider reducing intensity.
SELF-RESPECT on the line? Intensity should fit values.

2. CAPABILITY: Is person able to give me what I want? If YES, raise the intensity of ASKING.

Do I have what the person wants? If NO, raise the intensity of NO.

3. TIMELINESS: Is this a good time to ask? Is person "in the mood" for listening and paying attention to me? Am I catching person when he or she is likely to say yes to my request? If YES, raise the intensity of ASKING.

Is this a bad time to say no? Should I hold off answering for a while? If NO, raise the intensity of NO.

(cont.)

4. HOMEWORK: Have I done my homework? Do I know all the facts I need to know to support my request? Am I clear about what I want? If YES, raise the intensity of ASKING.

Is the other person's request clear? Do I know what I am agreeing to? If NO raise the intensity of NO.

5. AUTHORITY: Am I responsible for directing the person or telling the person what to do? If YES, raise the intensity of ASKING.

Does the person have authority over me (e.g., my boss, my teacher)? And is what the person is asking within his or her authority? If NO, raise the intensity of NO.

6. RIGHTS: Is person required by law or moral code to give me what I want? If YES, raise the intensity of ASKING.

Am I required to give the person what he or she wants? Would saying no violate the other person's rights? If NO, raise the intensity of NO.

7. RELATIONSHIP: Is what I want appropriate to the current relationship? If YES, raise the intensity of ASKING.

Is what the person asking for appropriate to our current relationship? If NO, raise the intensity of NO.

8. RECIPROCITY: What have I done for the person? Am I giving at least as much as I ask for? Am I willing to give if person says yes? If YES, raise the intensity of ASKING.

Do I owe person a favor? Does he or she do a lot for me? If NO, raise the intensity of NO.

9. LONG VERSUS SHORT TERM: Will being submissive (and not asking) get peace now but create problems in the long run? If YES, raise the intensity of ASKING.

Is giving in to get short-term peace more important than the long-term welfare of the relationship? Will I eventually regret or resent saying no? If NO, raise the intensity of NO.

10. RESPECT: Do I usually do things for myself? Am I careful to avoid acting helpless when I am not? If YES, raise the intensity of ASKING.

Will saying no make me feel bad about myself, even when I am thinking about it wisely? If NO, raise the intensity of NO.

Other factors: _____

_____

_____

Suggestions for Interpersonal
Effectiveness Practice

Interpersonal skills can only be learned if they are PRACTICED, PRACTICED, PRACTICED. To do this, you must be alert to every practice opportunity. If no situations arise naturally, then you may need to go out of your way to find or create opportunities to practice. Some of the following situations are examples of ones you can create for practice. Others are situations that may arise in your day-to-day life.

1. Go to a library and ask the librarian for assistance in finding a book. (Variation: ask salesperson to help you find something.)
2. While talking with someone, change the subject.
3. Invite a friend to dinner (at your house or at a restaurant).
4. Call an insurance company and ask about its rates.
5. Take old books to a used-book store and find out what they are worth. Leave after you have your information.
6. Pay for a newspaper, pack of gum, or anything else costing less than $.50 with a $5.00 bill.
7. In a drug store or candy store, ask for change for a $1.00 bill without buying anything.
8. Go to a luncheonette or lunch counter during a slack time and ask for a glass of water, drink it, say "Thank you," and walk out again.
9. Go into a restaurant and ask to use the restroom; leave without eating anything.
10. Phone the department of sanitation, ask to speak to the commissioner (or as highly placed an official as you can reach), and complain about the garbage collection in your neighborhood. (Variations on this theme are numerous—e.g., complaining about telephone service, newspaper delivery, taxi service, bus service, bad TV program, etc.)
11. Go to a full-service gas station and ask the attendant to check the water in your radiator (or air in your tires); leave without buying gas.
12. Get on a bus (or wait for a bus) and ask other passengers for change. (Variations on this theme are numerous—asking someone for change for a newspaper, parking meter, etc.)
13. Call and make an appointment to have your hair cut. Call back later and cancel the appointment. (Variations: Make and cancel dinner reservations; make and cancel airline reservations.)
14. Ask the pharmacist for information on an over-the-counter drug.
15. Ask for special "fixings" on a sandwich bought at McDonald's, Burger King, or another fast-food restaurant. A variation of this is to ask for a substitution on the menu when ordering a meal.
16. Ask a salesperson in a store to help you find something.
17. Ask the manager in the supermarket to order something that you would like to buy but the store doesn't now carry. *(cont.)*

18. Ask a clerk in the grocery store whether they have any fresher lettuce (or other fruit or vegetable) in the back of the store. (Variation: Ask the clerk to check whether an item you want is in the back if you don't find it on the shelf.)

19. Go to a deli counter and ask for 2 ounces of meat or cheese. Leave without buying anything else.

20. Go into a department store or gift store and ask the salesperson for help in choosing an item or a gift. (Variation: Ask salesperson for an opinion on outfit you are considering buying.)

21. Call and ask for information about jobs listed in the classified section of the newspaper. (Variations on this theme are numerous: Call about things being sold in the classified ads; call universities and ask for information about classes; etc.)

22. Ask coworkers or classmates to do a favor for you (e.g., fix you a cup of coffee while they are fixing their own, give you an opinion on some aspect of your work, etc.).

23. Ask someone for a ride.

24. Disagree with someone's opinion.

25. Express disagreement with a parent, spouse, partner, or close friend regarding specific topics (scheduling priorities, sexual practices, time spent together, etc.).

26. Express disagreement over social arrangements as planned by a parent, spouse, partner, or close friend.

27. Request parent, spouse, partner, or children to accept more responsibility in some specific area.

28. Ask a friend for help in fixing something.

29. Ask a person making too much noise to be a bit quieter (person talking in a movie, neighbor playing loud music, etc.).

30. Ask your therapist or counselor for a favor.

31. Ask for help in moving furniture.

32. Ask your landlord to fix leaky roof, faucet, broken appliances, creaky door, etc.

33. Go see a dentist or physician and tell him or her clearly what the problem is.

34. Order a nonalcoholic beverage in a bar or cocktail lounge.

35. Ask to be excused from class or ask to leave early.

36. Ask a person to stop doing something that bothers you.

37. Ask skills training leader (who is going overtime) to end the session because time is up.

38. Ask a teacher for time to speak to him or her and make a complaint or give a compliment about the class.

Other: _____

_____

_____

_____

INTERPERSONAL EFFECTIVENESS HANDOUT 8

Guidelines for Objectives Effectiveness: Getting What You Want

A way to remember these skills is to remember the term **"DEAR MAN."**

> **DESCRIBE**
> **EXPRESS**
> **ASSERT**
> **REINFORCE**
>
> (stay) **MINDFUL**
> **APPEAR CONFIDENT**
> **NEGOTIATE**

Describe

Describe the current SITUATION (if necessary).

Tell the person exactly what you are reacting to. Stick to the facts.

Express

Express your FEELINGS and OPINIONS about the situation.

Assume that your feelings and opinions are not self-evident. Give a brief rationale. Use phrases such as "I want," "I don't want," instead of "I need," "You should," or "I can't."

Assert

Assert yourself by ASKING for what you want or SAYING NO clearly.

Assume that others will not figure it out or do what you want unless you ask. Assume that others cannot read your mind. Don't expect others to know how hard it is for you to ask directly for what you want.

Reinforce

Reinforce or reward the person ahead of time by explaining CONSEQUENCES.

Tell the person the positive effects of getting what you want or need. Tell him or her (if necessary) the negative effects of your not getting it. Help the person feel good ahead of time for doing or accepting what you want. Reward him or her afterwards.

(cont.)

From *Skills Training Manual for Treating Borderline Personality Disorder* by Marsha Linehan. ©1993 The Guilford Press.

(stay) <u>M</u>indful	Keep your focus ON YOUR OBJECTIVES.
	Maintain your position. Don't be distracted.
"Broken record"	Keep asking, saying no, or expressing your opinion over and over and over.
Ignore	If another person attacks, threatens, or tries to change the subject, ignore the threats, comments, or attempts to divert you. Don't respond to attacks. Ignore distractions. Just keep making your point.
<u>A</u>ppear confident	Appear EFFECTIVE and competent.
	Use a confident voice tone and physical manner; make good eye contact. No stammering, whispering, staring at the floor, retreating, saying "I'm not sure," etc.
<u>N</u>egotiate	Be willing to GIVE TO GET. Offer and ask for alternative solutions to the problem. Reduce your request. Maintain no, but offer to do something else or to solve the problem another way. Focus on what will work.
Turn the tables	Turn the problem over to the other person. Ask for alternative solutions: "What do you think we should do?" "I'm not able to say yes, and you seem to really want me to. What can we do here?" "How can we solve this problem?"

Other ideas: _____

_____

_____

_____

_____

_____

_____

_____

_____

INTERPERSONAL EFFECTIVENESS HANDOUT 9

Guidelines for Relationship Effectiveness:
Keeping the Relationship

A way to remember these skills is to remember the word **"GIVE"** (DEAR MAN, GIVE):

(be) **GENTLE**

(act) **INTERESTED**

VALIDATE

(use an) **EASY MANNER**

(be) Gentle	Be COURTEOUS and temperate in your approach.
No attacks	No verbal or physical attacks. No hitting, clenching fists. Express anger directly.
No threats	No "manipulative" statements, no hidden threats. No "I'll kill myself if you. . . . " Tolerate a no to requests. Stay in the discussion even if it gets painful. Exit gracefully.
No judging	No moralizing. No "If you were a good person, you would. . . . " No " You should. . . . " "You shouldn't. . . . "
(act) Interested	LISTEN and be interested in the other person.
	Listen to the other person's point of view, opinion, reasons for saying no, or reasons for making a request of you. Don't interrupt, talk over, etc. Be sensitive to the person's desire to have the discussion at a later time. Be patient.
Validate	Validate or ACKNOWLEDGE the other person's feelings, wants, difficulties, and opinions about the situation. Be nonjudgmental out loud: "I can understand how you feel, but . . . "; "I realize this is hard for you, but . . . "; "I see that you are busy, and. . . . "
(use an) Easy manner	Use a little humor. SMILE. Ease the person along. Be light-hearted. Wheedle. Use a "soft sell" over a "hard sell." Be political.

Other ideas: _____

From *Skills Training Manual for Treating Borderline Personality Disorder* by Marsha Linehan. ©1993 The Guilford Press.

INTERPERSONAL EFFECTIVENESS HANDOUT 10

Guidelines for Self-Respect Effectiveness: Keeping Your Respect for Yourself

A way to remember these skills is to remember the word **"FAST"** (**DEAR MAN, GIVE FAST**).

> **(be) FAIR**
> **(no) APOLOGIES**
> **STICK TO VALUES**
> **(be) TRUTHFUL**

(be) Fair	Be fair to YOURSELF and to the OTHER person.
(no) Apologies	No OVERLY apologetic behavior. No apologizing for being alive, for making a request at all. No apologies for having an opinion, for disagreeing.
Stick to values	Stick to YOUR OWN values.
	Don't sell out your values or integrity for reasons that aren't very important. Be clear on what you believe is the moral or valued way of thinking and acting, and "stick" to your guns.
(be) Truthful	DON'T LIE, ACT HELPLESS when you are not, or EXAGGERATE. Don't make up excuses.

Other ideas: _____

_____

_____

_____

_____

_____

_____

_____

From *Skills Training Manual for Treating Borderline Personality Disorder* by Marsha Linehan. ©1993 The Guilford Press.

INTERPERSONAL EFFECTIVENESS
HOMEWORK SHEET 1

Goals and Priorities in Interpersonal Situations

Name _____ Date _____

Use this sheet to figure out your goals and priorities in any situation that creates a problem for you such as ones where: 1) your rights or wishes are not being respected, 2) you want someone to do or change something or give you something, 3) you want or need to say no or resist pressure to do something, 4) you want to get your position or point of view taken seriously, 5) there is confict with another person. Observe and describe in writing as close in time to the situation as possible. Write on back of page if you need more room.

PROMPTING EVENT for my problem: Who did what to whom? What led up to what?
What is it about this situation that is a problem for me?

My **WANTS AND DESIRES** in this situation:
OBJECTIVES: What specific results do I want? What changes do I want person to make?

RELATIONSHIP: How do I want the other person to feel about me after the interaction?

SELF-RESPECT: How do I want to feel about myself after the interaction?

My **PRIORITIES** in this situation: Rate priorities 1 (most important), 2 (second most important), or 3 (least important).

_____ OBJECTIVES   _____ RELATIONSHIP   _____ SELF-RESPECT

CONFLICTS IN PRIORITIES that make it hard to be effective in this situation?

From *Skills Training Manual for Treating Borderline Personality Disorder* by Marsha Linehan. ©1993 The Guilford Press.

INTERPERSONAL EFFECTIVENESS HOMEWORK SHEET 2

Observing and Describing Interpersonal Situations

Name _____ Date _____

Fill out this sheet during or just after a situation that creates a problem for you such as one where: 1) your rights or wishes are not being respected, 2) you want someone to do or change something or give you something, 3) you want or need to say no or resist pressure to do something, 4) you want to get your position or point of view taken seriously, 5) there is conflict with another person. Observe and describe in writing as close in time to the situation as possible. Write on back of page if you need more room.

PROMPTING EVENT for my problem? Who did what to whom? What led up to what?

What **I SAID OR DID** in the situation: (Be SPECIFIC.) Rate **INTENSITY** of response. (See p. 131.)

INTENSITY–RATING (0–6):_____

FACTORS REDUCING MY EFFECTIVENESS in this situation:
SKILLS LACKING: (What don't I know how to do or say?)

WORRY THOUGHTS:

EMOTIONS INTERFERING:

INDECISION (or conflict in goals) getting in the way:
OBJECTIVES: What results do I want? What changes do I want the person to make?

RELATIONSHIP: How do I want other person to feel about me after the interaction?

SELF-RESPECT: How do I want to feel about myself after the interaction?

CONFLICT or INDECISION?

ENVIRONMENTAL FACTORS getting in my way:

(cont.)

From *Skills Training Manual for Treating Borderline Personality Disorder* by Marsha Linehan. ©1993 The Guilford Press.

ASK?			**SAY NO?**	
:---:			:---:	
(If more YES's than NO's, ASK)			(If more NO's than YES's, say NO)	

YES NO Can person give me what I want?	**Capability**	Do I have what person wants?	YES NO
YES NO Good time for me to ask?	**Timeliness**	Is it a bad time for me to say no?	YES NO
YES NO Am I prepared?	**Homework**	Is request clear?	YES NO
YES NO Is what person does my business?	**Authority**	Is person in authority over me?	YES NO
YES NO Do I have a right to what I am asking for?	**Rights**	Does saying no violate person's rights?	YES NO
YES NO Is request appropriate to relationship?	**Relationship**	Is request appropriate?	YES NO
YES NO Am I asking less than I give?	**Reciprocity**	Does person give me a lot? Do I owe person?	YES NO
YES NO Is asking important to long-term goal?	**Goals**	Does no interfere with long-term goal?	YES NO
YES NO Am I acting competent?	**Respect**	Does wise mind say yes?	YES NO

_____ SUM of YES responses   SUM of NO responses _____

HIGH INTENSITY: TRY AND CHANGE THE SITUATION

Ask firmly, insist... **6** ...Refuse firmly, don't give in.

Ask firmly, resist no... **5** ...Refuse firmly, resist giving in.

Ask firmly, take no... **4** ...Refuse firmly, but reconsider.

Ask tentatively, take no... **3** ...Express unwillingness.

Hint openly, take no... **2** ...Express unwillingness, but say yes.

Hint indirectly, take no... **1** ...Express hesitancy, say yes.

Don't ask, don't hint... **0** ...Do what other wants without being asked.

LOW INTENSITY: ACCEPT THE SITUATION AS IT IS

Notes: _____

_____

_____

_____

_____

_____

INTERPERSONAL EFFECTIVENESS HOMEWORK SHEET 3

Using Interpersonal Effectiveness Skills

Name _____ Week Starting _____

Fill out this sheet whenever you practice your interpersonal skills and whenever you have an opportunity to practice even if you don't (or almost don't) do anything to practice. Write on back of page if you need more room.

PROMPTING EVENT for my problem: Who did what to whom? What led up to what?

OBJECTIVES IN SITUATION (What results I want):

RELATIONSHIP ISSUE (How I want other person to feel about me):

SELF-RESPECT ISSUE (How I want to feel about myself):

What **I SAID OR DID** in the situation: (Describe and check below.)

DEAR MAN (Getting what I want):

_____ Described situation?	_____ Mindful?
_____ Expressed feelings/opinions?	_____ Broken record?
_____ Asserted?	_____ Ignored attacks?
_____ Reinforced?	_____ Appeared confident?
	_____ Negotiated?

GIVE (Keeping the relationship):

_____ Gentle?	_____ Interested?
_____ No threats?	_____ Validated?
_____ No attacks?	_____ Easy manner?
_____ No judgments?	

FAST (Keeping my respect for myself):

_____ Fair?	_____ Stuck to values?
_____ (No) Apologies?	_____ Truthful?

INTENSITY OF MY RESPONSE (0–6): _____   **INTENSITY I WANTED** (0–6): _____

(cont.)

INTERPERSONAL EFFECTIVENESS HOMEWORK SHEET 3 (cont.)

FACTORS REDUCING MY EFFECTIVENESS (check and describe)

_____ SKILLS LACKING:

_____ WORRY THOUGHTS:

_____ EMOTIONS INTERFERING:

_____ INDECISION:

_____ ENVIRONMENT:

ASK?		SAY NO?	
(If more YES's than NO's, ASK)		(If more NO's than YES's, say NO)	
YES NO Can person give me what I want?	**Capability**	Do I have what person wants?	YES NO
YES NO Good time for me to ask?	**Timeliness**	Is it a bad time for me to say no?	YES NO
YES NO Am I prepared?	**Homework**	Is request clear?	YES NO
YES NO Is what person does my business?	**Authority**	Is person in authority over me?	YES NO
YES NO Do I have a right to what I am asking for?	**Rights**	Does saying no violate person's rights?	YES NO
YES NO Is request appropriate to relationship?	**Relationship**	Is request appropriate?	YES NO
YES NO Am I asking less than I give?	**Reciprocity**	Does person give me a lot? Do I owe person?	YES NO
YES NO Is asking important to long-term goal?	**Goals**	Does no interfere with long-term goal?	YES NO
YES NO Am I acting competent?	**Respect**	Does wise mind say yes?	YES NO

_____ SUM of YES responses   SUM of NO responses _____

HIGH INTENSITY: TRY AND CHANGE THE SITUATION

Ask firmly, insist... **6** ...Refuse firmly, don't give in.

Ask firmly, resist no... **5** ...Refuse firmly, resist giving in.

Ask firmly, take no... **4** ...Refuse firmly, but reconsider.

Ask tentatively, take no... **3** ...Express unwillingness.

Hint openly, take no... **2** ...Express unwillingness, but say yes.

Hint indirectly, take no... **1** ...Express hesitancy, say yes.

Don't ask, don't hint... **0** ...Do what other wants without being asked.

LOW INTENSITY: ACCEPT THE SITUATION AS IT IS

EMOTION REGULATION HANDOUT 1

Goals of Emotion Regulation Training

UNDERSTAND
EMOTIONS YOU EXPERIENCE

- Identify (observe and describe) emotion.

- Understand what emotions do for you.

REDUCE
EMOTIONAL VULNERABILITY

- Decrease negative vulnerability (vulnerability to emotion mind).

- Increase positive emotions.

DECREASE
EMOTIONAL SUFFERING

- Let go of painful emotions through mindfulness.

- Change painful emotions through opposite action.

EMOTION REGULATION HANDOUT 2

Myths about Emotions

1. There is a right way to feel in every situation.

   CHALLENGE: _____

2. Letting others know that I am feeling bad is weakness.

   CHALLENGE: _____

3. Negative feelings are bad and destructive.

   CHALLENGE: _____

4. Being emotional means being out of control.

   CHALLENGE: _____

5. Emotions can just happen for no reason.

   CHALLENGE: _____

6. Some emotions are really stupid.

   CHALLENGE: _____

7. All painful emotions are a result of a bad attitude.

   CHALLENGE: _____

8. If others don't approve of my feelings, I obviously shouldn't feel the way I do.

   CHALLENGE: _____

9. Other people are the best judge of how I am feeling.

   CHALLENGE: _____

10. Painful emotions are not really important and should be ignored.

    CHALLENGE: _____

11. _____

    CHALLENGE: _____

12. _____

    CHALLENGE: _____

13. _____

    CHALLENGE: _____

14. _____

    CHALLENGE: _____

15. _____

    CHALLENGE: _____

From *Skills Training Manual for Treating Borderline Personality Disorder* by Marsha Linehan. ©1993 The Guilford Press.

EMOTION REGULATION HANDOUT 3

Model for Describing Emotions

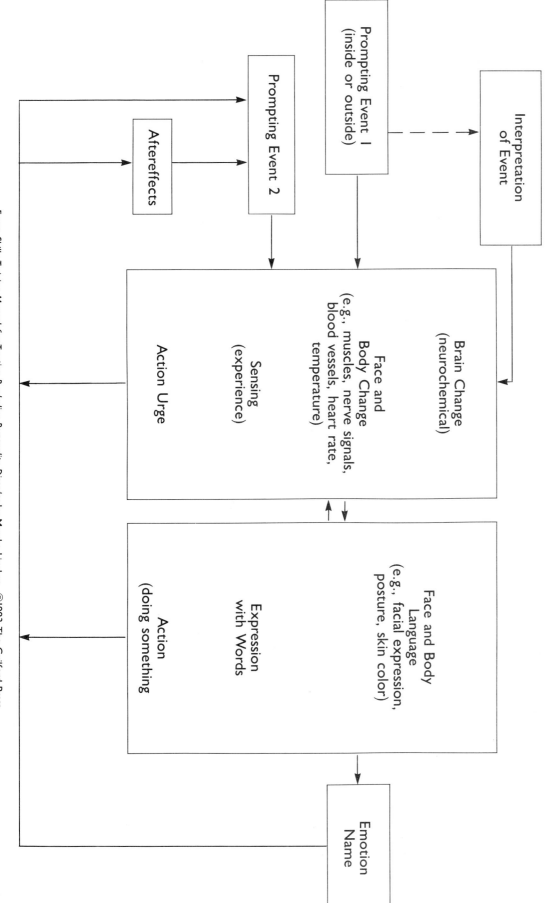

Ways to Describe Emotions

LOVE WORDS

love	compassion	longing
adoration	desire	lust
affection	enchantment	passion
arousal	fondness	sentimentality
attraction	infatuation	sympathy
caring	kindness	tenderness
charmed	liking	warm

Other: _____

_____

_____

_____

Prompting Events for Feeling Love

A person offers or gives you something you want, need, or desire.

A person does things you want or need the person to do.

You spend a lot of time with a person.

You share a special experience together with a person.

You have exceptionally good communication with a person.

Other: _____

_____

_____

_____

Interpretations That Prompt Feelings of Love

Believing that a person loves, needs, or appreciates you.

Thinking a person is physically attractive.

Judging a person's personality as wonderful, pleasing, or attractive.

Believing that a person can be counted on, will always be there for you.

Other: _____

_____

_____

_____

Experiencing the Emotion of Love

When with someone or thinking about someone:
    Feeling excited and full of energy.
    Fast heartbeat.
    Feeling and acting self-confident.
    Feeling invulnerable.
    Feeling happy, joyful, or exuberant.
    Feeling warm, trusting, and secure.
    Feeling relaxed and calm.
Wanting the best for a person.
Wanting to give things to a person.
Wanting to see and spend time with a person.
Wanting to spend your life with a person.
Wanting physical closeness or sex.
Wanting closeness.

Expressing and Acting on Love

Saying "I love you."
Expressing positive feelings to a person.
Eye contact, mutual gaze.
Touching, petting, hugging, holding, cuddling.
Smiling.
Sharing time and experiences with someone.
Doing things that the other person wants or needs.

Other: _____

_____

_____

_____

Aftereffects of Love

Only being able to see a person's positive side.
Feeling forgetful or distracted; daydreaming.
Feeling openness and trust.
Remembering other times and people you have loved.
Remembering other people who have loved you.
Remembering and imagining other positive events.

Other: _____

_____

_____

JOY WORDS

joy	enjoyment	glee	pride
amusement	enthrallment	happiness	rapture
bliss	enthusiasm	hope	relief
cheerfulness	euphoria	jolliness	satisfaction
contentment	excitement	joviality	thrill
delight	exhilaration	jubilation	triumph
eagerness	gaiety	optimism	zaniness
ecstasy	gladness	pleasure	zest
elation			zeal

Other: _____

_____

_____

_____

Prompting Events for Feeling Joy

Being successful at a task.

Achieving a desirable outcome.

Getting what you want.

Receiving esteem, respect, or praise.

Getting something you have worked hard for or worried about.

Receiving a wonderful surprise.

Things turning out better than you thought they would.

Reality exceeding your expectations.

Having very pleasurable sensations.

Doing things that create or bring to mind pleasurable sensations.

Being accepted by others.

Belonging (being around or in contact with people who accept you).

Receiving love, liking, or affection.

Being with or in contact with people who love or like you.

Other: _____

_____

_____

_____

EMOTION REGULATION HANDOUT 4 (cont.)

Interpretions That Prompt Feelings of Joy

Interpreting joyful events just as they are, without adding or subtracting.

Other: _____

_____

_____

_____

Experiencing the Emotion of Joy

Feeling excited.
Feeling physically energetic, active, or "hyper."
Feeling like giggling or laughing.
Feeling your face flush.

Expressing and Acting on Joy

Smiling.
Having a bright, glowing face.
Being bouncy or bubbly.
Communicating your good feelings.
Sharing the feeling.
Hugging people.
Jumping up and down.
Saying positive things.
Using an enthusiastic or excited voice.
Being talkative or talking a lot.

Other: _____

_____

_____

_____

Aftereffects of Joy

Being courteous or friendly to others.
Doing nice things for other people.
Having a positive outlook; seeing the bright side.
Having a high threshold for worry or annoyance.
Remembering and imagining other times you have felt joyful.
Expecting to feel joyful in the future.

Other: _____

_____

_____

From *Skills Training Manual for Treating Borderline Personality Disorder* by Marsha Linehan. ©1993 The Guilford Press.

ANGER WORDS

anger	disgust	grumpiness	rage
aggravation	dislike	hate	resentment
agitation	envy	hostility	revulsion
annoyance	exasperation	irritation	scorn
bitterness	ferocity	jealousy	spite
contempt	frustration	loathing	torment
cruelty	fury	mean-spiritedness	vengefulness
destructiveness	grouchiness	outrage	wrath

Other: _____

_____

_____

_____

Prompting Events for Feeling Anger

Losing power.

Losing status.

Losing respect.

Being insulted.

Not having things turn out the way you expected.

Experiencing physical pain.

Experiencing emotional pain.

Being threatened with physical or emotional pain by someone or something.

Having an important or pleasurable activity interrupted, postponed, or stopped.

Not obtaining something you want (which another person has).

Other: _____

_____

_____

_____

Interpretations That Prompt Feelings of Anger

Expecting pain.

Feeling that you have been treated unfairly.

Believing that things should be different.

Rigidly thinking "I'm right."

Judging that the situation is illegitimate, wrong, or unfair.

Ruminating about the event that set off the anger in the first place, or in the past.

Other: _____

_____

_____

_____

Experiencing the Emotion of Anger

Feeling incoherent.

Feeling out of control.

Feeling extremely emotional.

Feeling tightness or rigidity in your body.

Feeling your face flush or get hot.

Feeling nervous tension, anxiety or discomfort.

Feeling like you are going to explode.

Muscles tightening.

Teeth clamping together, mouth tightening.

Crying; being unable to stop tears.

Wanting to hit, bang the wall, throw something, blow up.

Other: _____

_____

_____

_____

Expressing and Acting on Anger

Frowning or not smiling; mean or unpleasant facial expression.

Gritting or showing your teeth in an unfriendly manner.

Grinning.

A red or flushed face.

Verbally attacking the cause of your anger; criticizing.

Physically attacking the cause of your anger.

Using obscenities or cursing.

Using a loud voice, yelling, screaming, or shouting.

Complaining or bitching; talking about how lousy things are.

Clenching your hands or fists.

Making aggressive or threatening gestures.

Pounding on something, throwing things, breaking things.

Walking heavily or stomping; slamming doors, walking out.

Brooding or withdrawing from contract with others.

Other: _____

_____

_____

_____

From *Skills Training Manual for Treating Borderline Personality Disorder* by Marsha Linehan. ©1993 The Guilford Press.

EMOTION REGULATION HANDOUT 4 (cont.)

Aftereffects of Anger

Narrowing of attention.

Attending only to the situation making you angry.

Ruminating about the situation making you angry and not being able to think of anything else.

Remembering and ruminating about other situations that have made you angry in the past.

Imagining future situations that will make you angry.

Depersonalization, dissociative experience, numbness.

Intense shame, fear, or other negative emotions.

Other: _____

_____

_____

_____

SADNESS WORDS

sadness	despair	grief	misery
agony	disappointment	homesickness	neglect
alienation	discontentment	hopelessness	pity
anguish	dismay	hurt	rejection
crushed	displeasure	insecurity	sorrow
defeat	distraught	isolation	suffering
dejection	gloom	loneliness	unhappiness
depression	glumness	melancholy	woe

Other: _____

_____

_____

_____

Prompting Events for Feeling Sadness

Things turning out badly.

Getting what you don't want.

Not getting what you want and believe you need in life; thinking about what you have not gotten that you wanted or needed.

Not getting what you have worked for.

Things being worse than you expected.

The death of someone you love; thinking about deaths of people you love.

Losing a relationship; thinking about losses.

Being separated from someone you care for or value; thinking about how much you miss someone.

From *Skills Training Manual for Treating Borderline Personality Disorder* by Marsha Linehan. ©1993 The Guilford Press.

Being rejected or excluded.
Being disapproved of or disliked; not being valued by people you care about.
Discovering that you are powerless or helpless.
Being with someone else who is sad, hurt or in pain.
Reading about other people's problems or troubles in the world.

Other: _____

_____

_____

_____

Interpretations That Prompt Feelings of Sadness

Believing that a separation from someone will last for a long time or will never end.
Believing that you are worthless or not valuable.
Believing that you will not get what you want or need in your life.
Hopeless beliefs.

Other: _____

_____

_____

_____

Experiencing the Emotion of Sadness

Feeling tired, run-down, or low in energy.
Feeling lethargic, listless; wanting to stay in bed all day.
Feeling as if nothing is pleasurable any more.
Feeling a pain or hollowness in your chest or gut.
Feeling empty.
Crying, tears, whimpering.
Feeling as if you can't stop crying, or feeling that if you ever start crying you will never
    be able to stop.
Difficulty swallowing.
Breathlessness.
Dizziness.

Other: _____

_____

_____

_____

EMOTION REGULATION HANDOUT 4 (cont.)

Expressing and Acting on Sadness

Frowning, not smiling.

Eyes drooping.

Sitting or lying around; being inactive.

Making slow, shuffling movements.

A slumped, drooping posture.

Withdrawing from social contact.

Talking little or not at all.

Using a low, quiet, slow, or monotonous voice.

Saying sad things.

Giving up and no longer trying to improve.

Moping, brooding, or acting moody.

Talking to someone about sadness.

Other: _____

_____

_____

_____

Aftereffects of Sadness

Feeling irritable, touchy, or grouchy.

Having a negative outlook; thinking only about the negative side of things.

Blaming or criticizing yourself.

Remembering or imagining other times you were sad and other losses.

Hopeless attitude.

Not being able to remember happy things.

Fainting spells.

Nightmares.

Insomnia.

Appetite disturbance, indigestion.

Yearning and searching for the thing lost.

Depersonalization, dissociative experiences, numbness, or shock.

Anger, shame, fear, or other negative emotions.

Other: _____

_____

_____

_____

From *Skills Training Manual for Treating Borderline Personality Disorder* by Marsha Linehan. ©1993 The Guilford Press.

FEAR WORDS

fear	fright	panic
apprehension	horror	shock
anxiety	hysteria	tenseness
distress	jumpiness	terror
dread	nervousness	uneasiness
edginess	overwhelmed	worry

Other: _____

_____

_____

_____

Prompting Events for Feeling Fear

Being in a new or unfamiliar situation.

Being alone (e.g., walking alone, being home alone, living alone).

Being in the dark.

Being in a situation where you have been threatened or gotten hurt in the past, or where painful things have happened.

Being in a situation somewhat like one where you were threatened or got hurt in the past, or where painful things have happened.

Being in situations where you have seen other people be threatened, get hurt, or have something painful happen.

Other: _____

_____

_____

_____

Interpretations That Prompt Feelings of Fear

Believing that someone might reject you, criticize, dislike, or disapprove of you.

Believing that failure is possible; expecting to fail.

Believing that you will not get help you want or believe you need.

Believing that you might lose help and assistance you already have.

Believing that you might lose someone or something you want.

Losing a sense of control; believing that you are helpless.

Losing a sense of mastery or competence.

Believing that you might be hurt or harmed, or that you might lose something valuable.

Believing that you might die, or that you are going to die.

Other: _____

_____

_____

_____

Experiencing the Emotion of Fear

Sweating or perspiring.

Feeling nervous, jittery, or jumpy.

Shaking, quivering, or trembling.

Darting eyes or quickly looking around.

Choking sensation, lump in throat.

Breathlessness, breathing fast.

Muscles tensing, cramping.

Diarrhea, vomiting.

Feeling of heaviness in stomach.

Getting cold.

Hair erect.

Other: _____

_____

_____

_____

Expressing and Acting on Fear

Engaging in nervous, fearful talk.

A shaky or trembling voice.

Crying or whimpering.

Screaming or yelling.

Pleading or crying for help.

Fleeing, running away.

Running or walking hurriedly.

Hiding from or avoiding what you fear.

Trying not to move.

Talking less or becoming speechless.

Frozen stare.

Others: _____

_____

_____

_____

Aftereffects of Fear

Losing your ability to focus or becoming disoriented.

Being dazed.

Losing control.

Remembering other threatening times, other times when things did not go well.

Imagining the possibility of more loss or failure.

Depersonalization, dissociative experiences, numbness, or shock.

Intense anger, shame, or other negative emotions.

Other: _____

_____

_____

SHAME WORDS

shame	discomposure	humiliation	mortification
contrition	embarrassment	insult	regret
culpability	guilt	invalidation	remorse

Other: _____

_____

_____

Prompting Events for Feeling Shame

Doing (feeling or thinking) something you (or people you admire) believe is wrong or immoral.

Being reminded of something wrong, immoral, or "shameful" you did in the past.

Exposure of a very private aspect of yourself or your life.

Having others find out that you have done something wrong.

Being laughed at, made fun of.

Being criticized in public, in front of someone else; remembering public criticism.

Others attacking your integrity.

Being betrayed by a person you love.

Being rejected by people you care about.

Failing at something you feel you are (or should be) competent to do.

Being rejected or criticized for something you expected praise for.

Having emotions that have been invalidated.

Other: _____

_____

_____

Interpretions That Prompt Feelings of Shame

Believing your body (or body part) is too big, too small, or not the right size.

Thinking that you are bad, immoral, or wrong.

Thinking that you have not lived up to your expectations of yourself.

Thinking that you have not lived up to other's expectations of you.

Thinking that your behavior, thoughts, or feelings are silly or stupid.

Judging yourself to be inferior, not "good enough," not as good as others.

Comparing yourself to others and thinking that you are a "loser."

Believing yourself unlovable.

Other: _____

_____

_____

Experiencing the Emotion of Shame

Pain in the pit of the stomach.

Sense of dread.

Crying, tears, sobbing.

Blushing, hot, red face.

Wanting to hide or cover your face.

Jitteriness, nervousness.

Choking sensation, suffocating.

Other: _____

_____

_____

Expressing and Acting on Shame

Withdrawing, covering the face, hiding.

Bowing your head, kneeling before the person, groveling.

Eyes down, darting eyes.

Avoiding the person you have harmed or the people who know you have done wrong.

Sinking back, slumped posture.

Saying you are sorry; apologizing.

Asking for forgiveness.

Giving gifts, trying to make up for the transgression.

Trying to repair the harm, fix up the damage, change the outcome.

Other: _____

_____

_____

Aftereffects of Shame

Avoiding thinking about your transgression, shutting down, blocking all emotions.

Engaging in distracting, impulsive behaviors to divert your mind or attention.

Believing you are defective.

Making resolutions to change.

Depersonalization, dissociative experiences, numbness, or shock.

Intense anger, sadness, fear, or other negative emotions.

Isolation, feeling alienated.

Other: _____

_____

_____

_____

OTHER IMPORTANT EMOTION WORDS

Interest, excitement, curiosity, pique, intrigue.

Weariness, dissatisfaction, disinclination.

Shyness, fragility, reserve, bashfulness, coyness, reticence.

Cautiousness, reluctance, suspiciousness, caginess, wariness.

Surprise, amazement, astonishment, awe, startle, wonder.

Boldness, bravery, courage, determination.

Powerfulness, a sense of competence, capability, mastery.

Dubiousness, skepticism, doubtfulness.

Apathy, boredom, dullness, ennui, fidgetiness, impatience, indifference, listlessness.

Other: _____

_____

_____

_____

Note. Selected emotional features were extracted from "Emotion Knowledge: Further Exploration of a Prototype Approach" by P. Shaver, J. Schwartz, D. Kirson, and C. O'Connor (1987). *Journal of Personality and Social Psychology, 52,* 1061–1086.

EMOTION REGULATION HANDOUT 5

What Good Are Emotions?

EMOTIONS COMMUNICATE TO (AND INFLUENCE) OTHERS.

- Facial expressions are a hard-wired part of emotions. In primitive societies and among animals, facial expressions communicate like words. Even in modern societies, facial expressions communicate faster than words.

- When it is important to us to communicate to others, or send them a message, it can be very hard for us to change our emotions.

- Whether we intend it or not, the communication of emotions influences others.

EMOTIONS ORGANIZE AND MOTIVATE ACTION.

- Emotions motivate our behavior. The action urge connected to specific emotions is often "hard-wired." Emotions prepare us for action.

- Emotions save time in getting us to act in important situations. We don't have to think everything through.

- Strong emotions help us overcome obstacles—in our mind and in the environment.

EMOTIONS CAN BE SELF-VALIDATING.

- Our emotional reactions to other people and to events can give us information about the situation. Emotions can be signals or alarms that something is happening.

- When this is carried to an extreme, emotions are treated as facts: "If I feel incompetent, I am." "If I get depressed when left alone, I shouldn't be left alone." "If I feel right about something, it is right." "If I'm afraid, it is threatening." "I love him, so he must be OK."

EMOTION REGULATION HANDOUT 6

Reducing Vulnerability to Negative Emotions: How to Stay Out of Emotion Mind

A way to remember these skills is to remember the term **"PLEASE MASTER."**

Treat PhysicaL illness
Balance Eating
Avoid mood-Altering drugs
Balance Sleep
Get Exercise
Build MASTERy

1. Treat PhysicaL illness: Take care of your body. See a doctor when necessary. Take prescribed medication.

2. Balance Eating: Don't eat too much or too little. Stay away from foods that make you feel overly emotional.

3. Avoid mood-Altering drugs: Stay off nonprescribed drugs, including alcohol.

4. Balance Sleep: Try to get the amount of sleep that helps you feel good. Keep to a sleep program if you are having difficulty sleeping.

5. Get Exercise: Do some sort of exercise every day; try to build up to 20 minutes of vigorous exercise.

6. Build MASTERy: Try to do one thing a day to make yourself feel competent and in control.

From *Skills Training Manual for Treating Borderline Personality Disorder* by Marsha Linehan. ©1993 The Guilford Press.

EMOTION REGULATION HANDOUT 7

Steps for Increasing Positive Emotions

BUILD POSITIVE EXPERIENCES

SHORT TERM: Do pleasant things that are possible now.

- INCREASE pleasant events that prompt positive emotions.
- Do ONE THING each day from the Adult Pleasant Events Schedule (see Emotion Regulation Handout 8)

LONG TERM: Make changes in your life so that positive events will occur more often. Build a "life worth living."

- Work toward goals: ACCUMULATE POSITIVES.
    Make list of positive events you want.
    List small steps toward goals.
    Take first step.
- ATTEND TO RELATIONSHIPS.
    Repair old relationships.
    Reach out for new relationships.
    Work on current relationships.
- AVOID AVOIDING. Avoid giving up.

BE MINDFUL OF POSITIVE EXPERIENCES

- FOCUS attention on positive events that happen.
- REFOCUS when your mind wanders to the negative.

BE UNMINDFUL OF WORRIES

DISTRACT from:

    Thinking about when the positive experience WILL END.
    Thinking about whether you DESERVE this positive experience.
    Thinking about how much more might be EXPECTED of you now.

From *Skills Training Manual for Treating Borderline Personality Disorder* by Marsha Linehan. ©1993 The Guilford Press.

EMOTION REGULATION HANDOUT 8

Adult Pleasant Events Schedule

1. Soaking in the bathtub
2. Planning my career
3. Getting out of (paying on) debt
4. Collecting things (coins, shells, etc.)
5. Going on vacation
6. Thinking how it will be when I finish school
7. Recycling old items
8. Going on a date
9. Relaxing
10. Going to a movie in the middle of the week
11. Jogging, walking
12. Thinking I have done a full day's work
13. Listening to music
14. Recalling past parties
15. Buying household gadgets
16. Lying in the sun
17. Planning a career change
18. Laughing
19. Thinking about my past trips
20. Listening to others
21. Reading magazines or newspapers
22. Hobbies (stamp collecting, model building, etc.)
23. Spending an evening with good friends
24. Planning a day's activities
25. Meeting new people
26. Remembering beautiful scenery
27. Saving money
28. Gambling
29. Going home from work
30. Eating
31. Practicing karate, judo, yoga
32. Thinking about retirement
33. Repairing things around the house
34. Working on my car (bicycle)
35. Remembering the words and deeds of loving people
36. Wearing sexy clothes
37. Having quiet evenings
38. Taking care of my plants
39. Buying, selling stock
40. Going swimming
41. Doodling
42. Exercising
43. Collecting old things
44. Going to a party
45. Thinking about buying things
46. Playing golf
47. Playing soccer
48. Flying kites
49. Having discussions with friends
50. Having family get-togethers
51. Riding a motorbike
52. Sex
53. Running track
54. Going camping
55. Singing around the house
56. Arranging flowers
57. Practicing religion (going to church, group praying, etc.)
58. Losing weight
59. Going to the beach
60. Thinking I'm an OK person
61. A day with nothing to do
62. Having class reunions

From *Skills Training Manual for Treating Borderline Disorder* by Marsha Linehan. ©1993 The Guilford Press.

63. Going skating
64. Going sailboating
65. Traveling abroad or in the United States
66. Painting
67. Doing something spontaneously
68. Doing needlepoint, crewel, etc.
69. Sleeping
70. Driving
71. Entertaining
72. Going to clubs (garden, Parents without Partners, etc.)
73. Thinking about getting married
74. Going hunting
75. Singing with groups
76. Flirting
77. Playing musical instruments
78. Doing arts and crafts
79. Making a gift for someone
80. Buying records
81. Watching boxing, wrestling
82. Planning parties
83. Cooking
84. Going hiking
85. Writing books (poems, articles)
86. Sewing
87. Buying clothes
88. Going out to dinner
89. Working
90. Discussing books
91. Sightseeing
92. Gardening
93. Going to the beauty parlor
94. Early morning coffee and newspaper
95. Playing tennis
96. Kissing
97. Watching my children (play)
98. Thinking I have a lot more going for me than most people
99. Going to plays and concerts
100. Daydreaming
101. Planning to go to school
102. Thinking about sex
103. Going for a drive
104. Listening to a stereo
105. Refinishing furniture
106. Watching TV
107. Making lists of tasks
108. Going bike riding
109. Walks in the woods (or at the waterfront)
110. Buying gifts
111. Traveling to national parks
112. Completing a task
113. Collecting shells
114. Going to a spectator sport (auto racing, horse racing)
115. Eating gooey, fattening foods
116. Teaching
117. Photography
118. Going fishing
119. Thinking about pleasant events
120. Staying on a diet
121. Playing with animals
122. Flying a plane
123. Reading fiction
124. Acting
125. Being alone
126. Writing diary entries or letters
127. Cleaning
128. Reading nonfiction
129. Taking children places

From *Skills Training Manual for Treating Borderline Personality Disorder* by Marsha Linehan. ©1993 The Guilford Press.

130. Dancing
131. Going on a picnic
132. Thinking "I did that pretty well" after doing something
133. Meditating
134. Playing volleyball
135. Having lunch with a friend
136. Going to the mountains
137. Thinking about having a family
138. Thoughts about happy moments in my childhood
139. Splurging
140. Playing cards
141. Solving riddles mentally
142. Having a political discussion
143. Playing softball
144. Seeing and/or showing photos or slides
145. Playing guitar
146. Knitting
147. Doing crossword puzzles
148. Shooting pool
149. Dressing up and looking nice
150. Reflecting on how I've improved
151. Buying things for myself (perfume, golf balls, etc.)
152. Talking on the phone
153. Going to museums
154. Thinking religious thoughts
155. Lighting candles
156. Listening to the radio
157. Getting a massage
158. Saying "I love you"
159. Thinking about my good qualities
160. Buying books
161. Taking a sauna or a steam bath
162. Going skiing
163. White-water canoeing
164. Going bowling
165. Doing woodworking
166. Fantasizing about the future
167. Taking ballet, tap dancing
168. Debating
169. Sitting in a sidewalk cafe
170. Having an aquarium
171. Erotica (sex books, movies)
172. Going horseback riding
173. Thinking about becoming active in the community
174. Doing something new
175. Making jigsaw puzzles
176. Thinking I'm a person who can cope

Other: _____

_____

_____

_____

_____

_____

_____

_____

_____

Note. Adapted from *The Adult Pleasant Events Schedule* by M. M. Linehan, E. Sharp, and A. M. Ivanoff, 1980, November, paper presented at the meeting of the Association for Advancement of Behavior Therapy, New York. Adapted by permissions of the authors.

EMOTION REGULATION HANDOUT 9

Letting Go of Emotional Suffering: Mindfulness of Your Current Emotion

---

OBSERVE YOUR EMOTION

- NOTE its presence.
- Step BACK.
- Get UNSTUCK from the emotion.

EXPERIENCE YOUR EMOTION

- As a WAVE, coming and going.

- Try not to BLOCK emotion.
- Try not to SUPPRESS emotion.

- Don't try to GET RID of emotion.
- Don't PUSH it away.

- Don't try to KEEP emotion around.
- Don't HOLD ON to it.
- Don't AMPLIFY it.

REMEMBER: YOU ARE NOT YOUR EMOTION

- Do not necessarily ACT on emotion.
- Remember times when you have felt DIFFERENT.

PRACTICE LOVING YOUR EMOTION

- Don't JUDGE your emotion.
- Practice WILLINGNESS.
- Radically ACCEPT your emotion.

From *Skills Training Manual for Treating Borderline Personality Disorder* by Marsha Linehan. ©1993 The Guilford Press.

EMOTION REGULATION HANDOUT 10

Changing Emotions by Acting Opposite to the Current Emotion

FEAR

- Do what you are afraid of doing . . . OVER AND OVER AND OVER.
- APPROACH events, places, tasks, activities, people you are afraid of.
- Do things to give yourself a sense of CONTROL and MASTERY.
- When overwhelmed, make a list of small steps or tasks you can do. DO THE FIRST THING on the list.

GUILT OR SHAME

When Guilt or Shame Is Justified
(Emotion fits your wise mind values):

- REPAIR the transgression.
  - Say you're sorry. APOLOGIZE.
  - MAKE THINGS BETTER; do something nice for person you offended (or for someone else if that is not possible).
- COMMIT to avoiding that mistake in the future.
- ACCEPT the consequences gracefully.
- Then LET IT GO.

When Guilt or Shame Is Unjustified
(Emotion does not fit your wise mind values):

- Do what makes you feel guilty or ashamed . . . OVER AND OVER AND OVER.
- APPROACH, don't avoid.

SADNESS OR DEPRESSION

- Get ACTIVE. APPROACH, don't avoid.
- Do things that make you feel COMPETENT AND SELF-CONFIDENT.

ANGER

- Gently AVOID person you are angry with rather than attacking. (Avoid thinking about him or her rather than ruminating.)
- Do something NICE rather than mean or attacking.
- Imagine SYMPATHY AND EMPATHY for other person rather than blame.

EMOTION REGULATION HOMEWORK SHEET 1

Observing and Describing Emotions

Name _____ Week Starting _____

Select a current or recent emotional reaction and fillout as much of this sheet as you can. If the prompting event for the emotion you are working on is another emotion that occured first (for example, feeling afraid prompted getting angry at yourself), then fill out a second homework sheet for that first emotion. Write on back of page if you need more room.

EMOTION NAMES: _____ _____ **INTENSITY** (0–100) _____

PROMPTING EVENT for my emotion: (who, what, when, where) What started the emotion?

_____

INTERPRETATIONS (beliefs, assumptions, appraisals) of the situation?

_____

BODY CHANGES and SENSING: What am I feeling in my body?

_____

BODY LANGUAGE What is my facial expression? posture? gestures?

_____

ACTION URGES: What do I feel like doing? What do I want to say?

_____

What **I SAID OR DID** in the situation: (Be specific)

_____

What **AFTER EFFECT** does the emotion have on me (my state of mind, other emotions, behavior, thoughts, memory, body, etc.)?

_____

| FUNCTION OF EMOTION: _____ |
| _____ |
| _____ |

EMOTION REGULATION HOMEWORK SHEET 2

Emotion Diary

Name _____ Week Starting _____

Record emotions (either the strongest emotion of the day, the longest-lasting one, or the one that was the most painful or gave you the most trouble). Analyze that emotion. Fill out an "OBSERVING AND DESCRIBING EMOTIONS" homework sheet if necessary, plus this diary sheet.

Day _____ Emotion _____ _____	Event	Emotion's function
Day _____ Emotion _____ _____	Event	Emotion's function
Day _____ Emotion _____ _____	Event	Emotion's function
Day _____ Emotion _____ _____	Event	Emotion's function
Day _____ Emotion _____ _____	Event	Emotion's function

From *Skills Training Manual for Treating Borderline Disorder* by Marsha Linehan. ©1993 The Guilford Press.

EMOTION REGULATION HOMEWORK SHEET 3

Steps for Reducing Painful Emotions

Name _____ Week starting _____

For each emotion regulation skill, check whether you used it during the week and describe what you did. Write on back of page if you need more room.

REDUCED VULNERABILITY TO EMOTION MIND: treated PhysicaL illness? _____

balanced Eating? _____

off mood-Altering drugs? _____

balanced Sleep? _____

Exercise? _____

MASTERy? _____

INCREASED POSITIVE EVENTS

INCREASED daily pleasant activities (circle):   M   T   W   TH   F   S   SUN (describe)

_____

LONG TERM GOALS worked on:

_____

ATTENDED TO RELATIONSHIPS? (describe)

_____

AVOIDED AVOIDING (describe)

MINDFULNESS OF POSITIVE EXPERIENCES THAT OCCURRED

_____ Focused (and refocused) attention on positive experiences?

_____ Distracted from worries about positive experiences?

MINDFULNESS OF THE CURRENT EMOTION

_____ Observed the emotion?   _____ Remembered:

_____ Experienced the emotion?   _____ Not to act on emotion?

_____ Times I've felt different?

OPPOSITE ACTION: How did I act opposite to current emotion?

DISTRESS TOLERANCE HANDOUT I

Crisis Survival Strategies

Skills for tolerating painful events and emotions when you cannot make things better right away.

DISTRACT with "Wise Mind ACCEPTS."

Activities
Contributing
Comparisons
Emotions
Pushing away
Thoughts
Sensations

SELF-SOOTHE the FIVE SENSES.

Vision
Hearing
Smell
Taste
Touch

IMPROVE THE MOMENT.

Imagery
Meaning
Prayer
Relaxation
One thing at a time
Vacation
Encouragement

PROS AND CONS

DISTRESS TOLERANCE HANDOUT I:
Crises Survival Strategies (cont.)

DISTRACTING

A useful way to remember these skills is the phrase
"Wise Mind ACCEPTS."

With **Activities:**

Engage in exercise or hobbies; do cleaning; go to events; call or visit a friend; play computer games; go walking; work; play sports; go out to a meal, have decaf coffee or tea; go fishing; chop wood, do gardening; play pinball.

With **Contributing:**

Contribute to someone; do volunteer work; give something to someone else; make something nice for someone else; do a surprising, thoughtful thing.

With **Comparisons:**

Compare yourself to people coping the same as you or less well than you. Compare yourself to those less fortunate than you. Watch soap operas; read about disasters, others' suffering.

With opposite **Emotions:**

Read emotional books or stories, old letters; go to emotional movies; listen to emotional music. *Be sure the event creates different emotions.* Ideas: scary movies, joke books, comedies, funny records, religious music, marching songs, "I Am Woman" (Helen Reddy); going to a store and reading funny greeting cards.

With **Pushing away:**

Push the situation away by leaving it for a while. Leave the situation mentally. Build an imaginary wall between yourself and the situation.

Or push the situation away by blocking it in your mind. Censor ruminating. Refuse to think about the painful aspects of the situation. Put the pain on a shelf. Box it up and put it away for a while.

With other **Thoughts:**

Count to 10; count colors in a painting or tree, windows, anything; work puzzles; watch TV; read.

With intense other **Sensations:**

Hold ice in hand; squeeze a rubber ball very hard; stand under a very hard and hot shower; listen to very loud music; sex; put rubber band on wrist, pull out, and let go.

From *Skills Training Manual for Treating Borderline Personality Disorder* by Marsha Linehan. ©1993 The Guilford Press.

DISTRESS TOLERANCE HANDOUT 1:
Crisis Survival Strategies (cont.)

SELF-SOOTHE

A way to remember these skills is to think of soothing each of your
FIVE SENSES:

With **Vision:**

Buy one beautiful flower; make one space in a room pretty; light a candle and watch the flame. Set a pretty place at the table, using your best things, for a meal. Go to a museum with beautiful art. Go sit in the lobby of a beautiful old hotel. Look at nature around you. Go out in the middle of the night and watch the stars. Walk in a pretty part of town. Fix your nails so they look pretty. Look at beautiful pictures in a book. Go to a ballet or other dance performance, or watch one on TV. Be mindful of each sight that passes in front of you, not lingering on any.

With **Hearing:**

Listen to beautiful or soothing music, or to invigorating and exciting music. Pay attention to sounds of nature (waves, birds, rainfall, leaves rustling). Sing to your favorite songs. Hum a soothing tune. Learn to play an instrument. Call 800 or other information numbers to hear a human voice. Be mindful of any sounds that come your way, letting them go in one ear and out the other.

With **Smell:**

Use your favorite perfume or lotions, or try them on in the store; spray fragrance in the air; light a scented candle. Put lemon oil on your furniture. Put potpourri in a bowl in your room. Boil cinnamon; bake cookies, cake, or bread. Smell the roses. Walk in a wooded area and mindfully breathe in the fresh smells of nature.

With **Taste:**

Have a good meal; have a favorite soothing drink such as herbal tea or hot chocolate (no alcohol); treat yourself to a dessert. Put whipped cream on your coffee. Sample flavors in an ice cream store. Suck on a piece of peppermint candy. Chew your favorite gum. Get a little bit of a special food you don't usually spend the money on, such as fresh-squeezed orange juice. Really taste the food you eat; eat one thing mindfully.

With **Touch:**

Take a bubble bath; put clean sheets on the bed. Pet your dog or cat. Have a massage; soak your feet. Put creamy lotion on your whole body. Put a cold compress on your forehead. Sink into a really comfortable chair in your home, or find one in a luxurious hotel lobby. Put on a silky blouse, dress, or scarf. Try on fur-lined gloves or fur coats in a department store. Brush your hair for a long time. Hug someone. Experience whatever you are touching; notice touch that is soothing.

From *Skills Training Manual for Treating Borderline Personality Disorder* by Marsha Linehan. ©1993 The Guilford Press.

DISTRESS TOLERANCE HANDOUT I:
Crisis Survival Strategies (cont.)

IMPROVE THE MOMENT

A way to remember these skills is the word
IMPROVE.

With **Imagery:**

Imagine very relaxing scenes. Imagine a secret room within yourself, seeing how it is decorated. Go into the room whenever you feel very threatened. Close the door on anything that can hurt you. Imagine everything going well. Imagine coping well. Make up a fantasy world that is calming and beautiful and let your mind go with it. Imagine hurtful emotions draining out of you like water out of a pipe.

With **Meaning:**

Find or create some purpose, meaning, or value in the pain. Remember, listen to, or read about spiritual values. Focus on whatever positive aspects of a painful situation you can find. Repeat them over and over in your mind. Make lemonade out of lemons.

With **Prayer:**

Open your heart to a supreme being, greater wisdom, God, your own wise mind. Ask for strength to bear the pain in this moment. Turn things over to God or a higher being.

With **Relaxation:**

Try muscle relaxing by tensing and relaxing each large muscle group, starting with your hands and arms, going to the top of your head, and then working down; listen to a relaxation tape; exercise hard; take a hot bath or sit in a hot tub; drink hot milk; massage your neck and scalp, your calves and feet. Get in a tub filled with very cold or hot water and stay in it until the water is tepid. Breathe deeply; half-smile; change facial expression.

With **One thing in the moment:**

Focus your entire attention on just what you are doing right now. Keep yourself in the very moment you are in; put your mind in the present. Focus your entire attention on physical sensations that accompany nonmental tasks (e.g. walking, washing, doing dishes, cleaning, fixing). Be aware of how your body moves during each task. Do awareness exercises.

DISTRESS TOLERANCE HANDOUT I:
Crisis Survival Strategies (cont.)

With a brief **Vacation:**

Give yourself a brief vacation. Get in bed and pull the covers up over your head for 20 minutes. Rent a motel room at the beach or in the woods for a day or two; drop your towels on the floor after you use them. Ask your roommate to bring you coffee in bed or make you dinner (offer to reciprocate). Get a schlocky magazine or newspaper at the grocery store, get in bed with chocolates, and read it. Make yourself milk toast, bundle up in a chair, and eat it slowly. Take a blanket to the park and sit on it for a whole afternoon. Unplug your phone for a day, or let your answering machine screen your calls. Take a 1-hour breather from hard work that must be done.

With **Encouragement:**

Cheerlead yourself. Repeat over and over: "I can stand it," "It won't last forever," "I will make it out of this," I'm doing the best I can do."

Thinking of PROS AND CONS

Make a list of the pros and cons of *tolerating* the distress. Make another list of the pros and cons of *not tolerating* the distress—that is, of coping by hurting yourself, abusing alcohol or drugs, or doing something else impulsive.

Focus on long-term goals, the light at the end of the tunnel. Remember times when pain has ended.

Think of the positive consequences of tolerating the distress. Imagine in your mind how good you will feel if you achieve your goals, if you don't act impulsively.

Think of all of the negative consequences of not tolerating your current distress. Remember what has happened in the past when you have acted impulsively to escape the moment.

From *Skills Training Manual for Treating Borderline Personality Disorder* by Marsha Linehan. ©1993 The Guilford Press.

DISTRESS TOLERANCE HANDOUT 2

Guidelines for Accepting Reality: Observing-Your-Breath Exercises

OBSERVING YOUR BREATH:

Focus your attention on your breath, coming in and out. Observe your breathing as a way to center yourself in your wise mind. Observe your breathing as a way to take hold of your mind, dropping off nonacceptance and fighting reality.

I. DEEP BREATHING

Lie on your back. Breathe evenly and gently, focusing your attention on the movement of your stomach. As you begin to breathe in, allow your stomach to rise in order to bring air into the lower half of your lungs. As the upper halves of your lungs begin to fill with air, your chest begins to rise and your stomach begins to lower. Don't tire yourself. Continue for 10 breaths. The exhalation will be longer that the inhalation.

2. MEASURING YOUR BREATH BY YOUR FOOTSTEPS

Walk slowly in a yard, along a sidewalk, or on a path. Breathe normally. Determine the length of your breath, the exhalation and the inhalation, by the number of your footsteps. Continue for a few minutes. Begin to lengthen your exhalation by one step. Do not force a longer inhalation. Let it be natural. Watch your inhalation carefully to see whether there is a desire to lengthen it. Continue for 10 breaths.

Now lengthen the exhalation by one more footstep. Watch to see whether the inhalation also lengthens by one step or not. Only lengthen the inhalation when you feel that it will give delight. After 20 breaths, return your breath to normal. About 5 minutes later, you can begin the practice of lengthened breaths again. When you feel the least bit tired, return to normal. After several sessions of the practice of lengthened breath, your exhalation and inhalation will grow equal in length. Do not practice long, equal breaths for more than 10 to 20 breaths before returning to normal.

3. COUNTING YOUR BREATH

Sit cross-legged on the floor (sit in the half or full lotus position if you know how); or sit in a chair with your feet on the floor; or kneel; or lie flat on the floor; or take a walk. As you inhale, be aware that "I am inhaling, 1." When you exhale, be aware that "I am exhaling, 1." Remember to breathe from the stomach. When beginning the second inhalation, be aware that "I am inhaling, 2." And slowly exhaling, be aware that "I am exhaling, 2." Continue on up through 10. After you have reached 10, return to 1. Whenever you lose count, return to 1.

(cont.)

4. FOLLOWING YOUR BREATH WHILE LISTENING TO MUSIC

Listen to a piece of music. Breathe long, light, and even breaths. Follow your breath; be master of it while remaining aware of the movement and sentiments of the music. Do not get lost in the music, but continue to be master of your breath and yourself.

5. FOLLOWING YOUR BREATH WHILE CARRYING ON A CONVERSATION

Breathe long, light, and even breaths. Follow your breath while listening to a friend's words and to your own replies. Continue as with the music.

6. FOLLOWING THE BREATH

Sit cross-legged on the floor (sit in the half or full lotus position if you know how); or sit in a chair with your feet on the floor; or kneel; or lie flat on the floor; or take a walk. Begin to inhale gently and normally (from the stomach), aware that "I am inhaling normally." Exhale in awareness, "I am exhaling normally." Continue for three breaths. On the fourth breath, extend the inhalation, aware that "I am breathing in a long inhalation." Exhale in awareness, "I am breathing out a long exhalation." Continue for three breaths.

Now follow your breath carefully, aware of every movement of your stomach and lungs. Follow the entrance and exit of air. Be aware that "I am inhaling and following the inhalation from its beginning to its end. I am exhaling and following the exhalation from its beginning to its end."

Continue for 20 breaths. Return to normal. After 5 minutes, repeat the exercise. Maintain a half-smile while breathing. Once you have mastered this exercise, move on to the next.

7. BREATHING TO QUIET THE MIND AND BODY

Sit cross-legged on the floor (sit in half or full lotus position if you know how); or sit in a chair with your feet on the floor; or kneel; or lie flat on the floor. Half-smile. Follow your breath. When your mind and body are quiet, continue to inhale and exhale very lightly; be aware that "I am breathing in and making the breath and body light and peaceful. I am exhaling and making the breath and body light and peaceful." Continue for three breaths, giving rise to the thought, "I am breathing in while my body and mind are at peace. I am breathing out while my body and mind are at peace."

Maintain this thought in awareness from 5 to 30 minutes, according to your ability and to the time available to you. The beginning and end of the practice should be relaxed and gentle. When you want to stop, gently massage the muscles in your legs before returning to a normal sitting position. Wait a moment before standing up.

Note. Adapted from *The Miracle of Mindfulness: A Manual of Meditation* (pp. 81–84) by Thich Nhat Hanh, 1976, Boston: Beacon Press. Copyright 1987 by Mobi Ho. Adapted by permission.

DISTRESS TOLERANCE HANDOUT 3

Guidelines for Accepting Reality: Half-Smiling Exercises

HALF-SMILE

Accept reality with your body. *Relax (by letting go or by just tensing and then letting go) your face, neck, and shoulder muscles and half-smile with your lips.* A tense smile is a grin (and might tell the brain you are hiding or masking). A half-smile is slightly up-turned lips with a relaxed face. Try to adopt a serene facial expression. Remember, your body communicates to your mind.

1. HALF-SMILE WHEN YOU FIRST AWAKE IN THE MORNING

Hang a branch, any other sign, or even the word "smile" on the ceiling or wall so that you see it right away when you open your eyes. This sign will serve as your reminder. Use these seconds before you get out of bed to take hold of your breath. Inhale and exhale three breaths gently while maintaining a half-smile. Follow your breaths.

2. HALF-SMILE DURING YOUR FREE MOMENTS

Anywhere you find yourself sitting or standing, half-smile. Look at a child, a leaf, a painting on a wall, or anything that is relatively still, and smile. Inhale and exhale quietly three times.

3. HALF-SMILE WHILE LISTENING TO MUSIC

Listen to a piece of music for 2 or 3 minutes. Pay attention to the words, music, rhythm, and sentiments of the music you are listening to (not your daydreams of other times). Half-smile while watching your inhalations and exhalations.

4. HALF-SMILE WHEN IRRITATED

When you realize "I'm irritated," half-smile at once. Inhale and exhale quietly, maintaining a half-smile for three breaths.

5. HALF-SMILE IN A LYING-DOWN POSITION

Lie on your back on a flat surface without the support of mattress or pillow. Keep your two arms loosely by your sides and keep your two legs slightly apart, stretched out before you. Maintain a half-smile. Breathe in and out gently, keeping your attention focused on your breath. Let go of every muscle in your body. Relax each muscle as though it were sinking down through the floor, or as though it were as soft and yielding as a piece of silk hanging in the breeze to dry. Let go entirely, keeping your attention only on your breath and half-smile. Think of yourself as a cat, completely relaxed before a warm fire, whose muscles yield without resistance to anyone's touch. Continue for 15 breaths.

(cont.)

From *Skills Training Manual for Treating Borderline Personality Disorder* by Marsha Linehan. ©1993 The Guilford Press.

6. HALF-SMILE IN A SITTING POSITION

Sit on the floor with your back straight, or on a chair with your two feet touching the floor. Half-smile. Inhale and exhale while maintaining the half-smile. Let go.

7. HALF-SMILE WHILE CONTEMPLATING THE PERSON YOU HATE OR DESPISE THE MOST

Sit quietly. Breathe and smile a half-smile. Imagine the image of the person who has caused you the most suffering. Regard the features you hate or despise the most or find the most repulsive. Try to examine what makes this person happy and what causes suffering in his or her daily life. Imagine the person's perceptions; try to see what patterns of thought and reason this person follows. Examine what motivates this person's hopes and actions. Finally, consider the person's consciousness. See whether the person's views and insights are open and free or not, and whether or not the person has been influenced by any prejudices, narrow-mindedness, hatred, or anger. See whether or not the person is master of himself or herself. Continue until you feel compassion rise in your heart like a well filling with fresh water, and your anger and resentment disappear. Practice this exercise many times on the same person.

Notes/Other times to half-smile: _____

_____

_____

_____

_____

_____

_____

_____

_____

_____

_____

_____

_____

Note. Adapted from *The Miracle of Mindfulness: A Manual on Meditation* (pp. 77–81, 93) by Thich Nhat Hanh, 1976, Boston: Beacon Press. Copyright 1976 by Thich Nhat Hanh. Adapted by permission.

DISTRESS TOLERANCE HANDOUT 4

Guidelines for Accepting Reality: Awareness Exercises

1. AWARENESS OF THE POSITIONS OF THE BODY

This can be practiced in any time and place. Begin to focus your attention on your breath. Breathe quietly and more deeply than usual. Be mindful of the position of your body, whether you are walking, standing, lying, or sitting down. Know where you walk, stand, lie, or sit. Be aware of the purpose of your position. For example, you might be conscious that you are standing on a green hillside in order to refresh yourself, to practice breathing, or just to stand. If there is no purpose, be aware that there is no purpose.

2. AWARENESS OF CONNECTION TO THE UNIVERSE

This can be practiced any time, any place. Focus your attention on where your body touches an object (floor or ground, air molecules, a chair or arm rest, your bed sheets and covers, your clothes, etc.). Try to see all the ways you are connected to and accepted by that object. Consider the function of that object with relation to you. That is, consider what the object does for you. Consider its kindness in doing that. Experience the sensation of touching the object and focus your entire attention on that kindness until a sense of being connected or loved or cared for arises in your heart.

Examples: Focus your attention on your feet touching the ground. Consider the kindness of the ground holding you up, providing a path for you to get to other things, not letting you fall away from everything else. Focus your attention on your body touching the chair you sit in. Consider how the chair accepts you totally, holds you up, supports your back, keeps you from falling down on the floor. Focus your attention on the sheets and covers on your bed. Consider the touch of the sheets and covers holding you, surrounding and keeping you warm and comfortable. Consider the walls in the room. They keep out the wind and the cold and the rain. Think of how the walls are connected to you via the floor and the air in the room. Experience your connection to the walls that provide you with a secure place to do things. Go hug a tree. Think of how you and the tree are connected. Life is in you and in the tree and both of you are warmed by the sun, held by the air and supported by the earth. Try and experience the tree loving you by providing something to lean on, or by shading you.

3. AWARENESS WHILE MAKING TEA OR COFFEE

Prepare a pot of tea or coffee to serve a guest or to drink by yourself. Do each movement slowly, in awareness. Do not let one detail of your movements go by without being aware of it. Know that your hand lifts the pot by its handle. Know that you are pouring the fragrant, warm tea or coffee into the cup. Follow each step in awareness. Breathe gently and more deeply than usual. Take hold of your breath if your mind strays.

4. AWARENESS WHILE WASHING THE DISHES

Wash the dishes consciously, as though each bowl is an object of contemplation. Consider each bowl as sacred. Follow your breath to prevent your mind from straying. Do not try to hurry to get the job over with. Consider washing the dishes the most important thing in life.

5. AWARENESS WHILE HAND-WASHING CLOTHES

Do not wash too many clothes at one time. Select only three or four articles of clothing. Find the most comfortable position to sit or stand so as to prevent a backache. Scrub the clothes consciously. Hold your attention on every movement of your hands and arms. Pay attention to the soap and water. When you have finished scrubbing and rinsing, your mind and body will feel as clean and fresh as your clothes. Remember to maintain a half-smile and take hold of your breath whenever your mind wanders.

6. AWARENESS WHILE CLEANING HOUSE

Divide your work into stages: straightening things and putting away books, scrubbing the toilet, scrubbing the bathroom, sweeping the floors, and dusting. Allow a good length of time for each task. Move slowly, three times more slowly than usual. Focus your attention fully on each task. For example, while placing a book on the shelf, look at the book, be aware of what book it is, know that you are in the process of placing it on the shelf, and know that you intend to put it in that specific place. Know that your hand reaches for the book, and picks it up. Avoid any abrupt or harsh movement. Maintain awareness of the breath, especially when your thoughts wander.

7. AWARENESS WHILE TAKING A SLOW-MOTION BATH

Allow yourself 30 to 45 minutes to take a bath. Don't hurry for even a second. From the moment you prepare the bath water to the moment you put on clean clothes, let every motion be light and slow. Be attentive of every movement. Place your attention to every part of your body, without discrimination or fear. Be aware of each stream of water on your body. By the time you've finished, your mind will feel as peaceful and light as your body. Follow your breath. Think of yourself as being in a clean and fragrant lotus pond in the summer.

8. PRACTICING AWARENESS WITH MEDITATION

Sit comfortably on the floor with your back straight, on the floor or in a chair with both feet touching the floor. Close your eyes all the way, or open them slightly and gaze at something near. With each breath, say to yourself, quietly and gently, the word "One." As you inhale, say the word "One." As you exhale, say the word "One," calmly and slowly. Try to collect your whole mind and put it into this one word. When your mind strays, return gently to saying "One." *If you start wanting to move, try not to move. Just gently observe wanting to move. Continue practicing a little past wanting to stop. Just gently observe wanting to stop.*

Note. Exercises 1 and 3–8 are adapted from *The Miracle of Mindfulness: A Manual on Meditation* (pp. 84–87) by Thich Nhat Hanh, 1976, Boston: Beacon Press. Copyright 1976 by Thich Nhat Hanh. Adapted by permission.

DISTRESS TOLERANCE HANDOUT 5

Basic Principles of Accepting Reality

RADICAL ACCEPTANCE

- Freedom from suffering requires ACCEPTANCE from deep within of what is. Let yourself go completely with what is. Let go of fighting reality.

- ACCEPTANCE is the only way out of hell.

- Pain creates suffering only when you refuse to ACCEPT the pain.

- Deciding to tolerate the moment is ACCEPTANCE.

- ACCEPTANCE is acknowledging what is.

- To ACCEPT something is not the same as judging it good.

TURNING THE MIND

- Acceptance of reality as it is requires an act of CHOICE. It is like coming to a fork in the road. You have to turn your mind towards the acceptance road and away from the "rejecting reality" road.

- You have to make an inner COMMITMENT to accept.

  The COMMITMENT to accept does not itself equal acceptance. It just turns you toward the path. But it is the first step.

  You have to turn your mind and commit to acceptance OVER AND OVER AND OVER again. Sometimes, you have to make the commitment many times in the space of a few minutes.

WILLINGNESS

Cultivate a WILLING response to each situation.

- Willingness is DOING JUST WHAT IS NEEDED in each situation, in an unpretentious way. It is focusing on effectiveness.

- Willingness is listening very carefully to your WISE MIND, acting from your inner self.

- Willingness is ALLOWING into awareness your connection to the universe— to the earth, to the floor you are standing on, to the chair you are sitting on, to the person you are talking to.

(over) WILLFULNESS

Replace WILLFULNESS with WILLINGNESS.

- Willfulness is SITTING ON YOUR HANDS when action is needed, refusing to make changes that are needed.

- Willfulness is GIVING UP.

- Willfulness is the OPPOSITE OF "DOING WHAT WORKS," being effective.

- Willfulness is trying to FIX every situation.

- Willfulness is REFUSING TO TOLERATE the moment.

DISTRESS TOLERANCE HOMEWORK SHEET I

Crises Survival Strategies

Name _____ Week starting _____

For each survival skill, check whether you used it during the week and write down your level of distress tolerance both before (pre) and after (post) using the strategy as follows: 0 = "No tolerance, a nightmare" to 100 = "Easy tolerance, piece of cake." List what you tried specifically on the back side of this sheet.

Skill	Mon Pre/ Post	Tues Pre/ Post	Wed Pre/ Post	Thur Pre/ Post	Fri Pre/ Post	Sat Pre/ Post	Sun Pre/ Post
DISTRACTING: "Wise Mind ACCEPTS"							
Activities	/	/	/	/	/	/	/
Contributions	/	/	/	/	/	/	/
Comparisons	/	/	/	/	/	/	/
Emotions	/	/	/	/	/	/	/
Pushing away	/	/	/	/	/	/	/
Thoughts	/	/	/	/	/	/	/
Sensations	/	/	/	/	/	/	/
SELF-SOOTHING: the five senses							
Vision	/	/	/	/	/	/	/
Hearing	/	/	/	/	/	/	/
Smell	/	/	/	/	/	/	/
Taste	/	/	/	/	/	/	/
Touch	/	/	/	/	/	/	/
IMPROVING THE MOMENT: IMPROVE							
Imagery	/	/	/	/	/	/	/
Meaning	/	/	/	/	/	/	/
Prayer	/	/	/	/	/	/	/
Relaxation	/	/	/	/	/	/	/
One thing in the moment	/	/	/	/	/	/	/
Vacation	/	/	/	/	/	/	/
Encouragement	/	/	/	/	/	/	/
Thinking of PROS & CONS	/	/	/	/	/	/	/

(cont.)